Pediatric Intensive Care Protocol

Pediatric Intensive Care Protocol

Santosh T Soans MBBS MD DCH (Pediatric Intensivist)
Professor and Head
Department of Pediatrics
AJ Institute of Medical Sciences
Mangalore, Karnataka, India

Arun MK MD (Pediatrics) DNB (Pediatrics)
Assistant Professor
Kasturba Medical College
Mangalore, Karnataka, India

JAYPEE BROTHERS MEDICAL PUBLISHERS (P) LTD

Bengaluru • New Delhi • St Louis (USA) • Panama City (Panama) • Ahmedabad
Chennai • Hyderabad • Kochi • Kolkata • Lucknow • Mumbai • Nagpur

Published by
Jitendar P Vij
Jaypee Brothers Medical Publishers (P) Ltd

Corporate Office
4838/24 Ansari Road, Daryaganj, **New Delhi** - 110002, India
Phone: +91-11-43574357, Fax: +91-11-43574314

Registered Office
B-3 EMCA House, 23/23B Ansari Road, Daryaganj, **New Delhi** - 110 002, India
Phones: +91-11-23272143, +91-11-23272703, +91-11-23282021
+91-11-23245672, Rel: +91-11-32558559, Fax: +91-11-23276490, +91-11-23245683
e-mail: jaypee@jaypeebrothers.com, Website: www.jaypeebrothers.com

Offices in India

- **Ahmedabad**, Phone: Rel: +91-79-32988717, e-mail: ahmedabad@jaypeebrothers.com
- **Bengaluru**, Phone: Rel: +91-80-32714073, e-mail: bangalore@jaypeebrothers.com
- **Chennai**, Phone: Rel: +91-44-32972089, e-mail: chennai@jaypeebrothers.com
- **Hyderabad**, Phone: Rel:+91-40-32940929, e-mail: hyderabad@jaypeebrothers.com
- **Kochi**, Phone: +91-484-2395740, e-mail: kochi@jaypeebrothers.com
- **Kolkata**, Phone: +91-33-22276415, e-mail: kolkata@jaypeebrothers.com
- **Lucknow**, Phone: +91-522-3040554, e-mail: lucknow@jaypeebrothers.com
- **Mumbai**, Phone: Rel: +91-22-32926896, e-mail: mumbai@jaypeebrothers.com
- **Nagpur**, Phone: Rel: +91-712-3245220, e-mail: nagpur@jaypeebrothers.com

Overseas Offices

- **North America Office, USA,** Ph: 001-636-6279734
  e-mail: jaypee@jaypeebrothers.com, anjulav@jaypeebrothers.com
- **Central America Office, Panama City, Panama,** Ph: 001-507-317-0160
  e-mail: cservice@jphmedical.com, Website: www.jphmedical.com

Pediatric Intensive Care Protocol

First Edition : **2010**

ISBN 978-81-8448-867-8

Typeset at JPBMP typesetting unit

Printed at

Dedicated to

Our parents who have helped and guided us
during the most difficult times of
our medical education

Preface

This book is intended for all those working in the Pediatric Intensive Care Unit. Pediatrics is now blooming from its budding state. The wealth of existing and new information in pediatric intensive care and the need for a comprehensive book has prompted the evolution of this book.

In the field of pediatric intensive care, plenty of information are available, but they are scattered in segments. We have assimilated and compiled this comprehensive guide to evaluate and manage pediatric intensive care.

The hours spent on call by postgraduates students are usually thought to be stressful, exhausting and overwhelming. While this is frequently true, we believe that time spent on call is extremely valuable part of overall education of the physician in training. Evaluating and managing problems that arise in emergencies when immediate help from attending consultants may not be available encourages independent thinking, clinical reasoning and decision-making. In addition, the successful management of these problems builds confidence and offers postgraduates an opportunity to test their skills and develop their knowledge base.

Learning to manage acute problems when on call, especially very sick children in intensive care is heavily dependent on experience. There may be a great deal of uncertainty. It is at times like these that ready reference is of immense help in managing crisis. This book is both concise and thorough. It spares the pediatrician great detail usually found in textbooks. We are sure it is going to be helpful to postgraduates as well as practicing pediatricians.

Santosh T Soans
Arun MK

Acknowledgments

Bringing out a well-researched book like this is never an easy task and many people have helped in their own ways and made it possible for this book to see the light of this day. We hereby wish to acknowledge few of our colleagues and friends who have provided me help, inspiration and motivation—Dr Sanjeeva Rai, Dr Subba Rao, Dr Prakash Saldhana, Dr Habib Khan, Dr Ramesh Pai, Dr Naveen Benakappa and Dr Dinesh SR. We also acknowledge the help given by the postgraduates of our institution during this time.

Contents

1

Basic Life Support

The following points should be considered while attending to a child with suspected cardiorespiratory arrest.

- The American heart association advocates 'phone first' approach to irresponsive adult, which is designed to bring defibrillation facility as quickly as possible. In pediatric age group, 1 minute of BLS to be done before leaving the unresponsive child to activate Emergency Medical Services (EMS) ('Phone fast' approach).

  If 2 rescuers are present CPR and activation of emergency system are done simultaneously. If alone and cause of emergency known, you can provide targeted response. When cause of emergency is not known for infants and children < 8 yrs—provide CPR first and then phone fast, because respiratory cause of arrest is more common.

  Children > 8 yrs – phone first and then provide CPR because cardiac cause of arrest more common (Exception—submersion, trauma, drug overdose).
- Ensure safety of rescuer and victim. Follow universal precautions.
- Stimulate—stimulate gently and avoid shaking the victim or moving if trauma is suspected.

- Tongue is the most common cause of airway obstruction in an unconscious child.
- Maneuvers to open airway are designed to lift the tongue away from back of pharynx; head tilt-chin lift or jaw thrust, maneuvers.
- When head and neck injury is suspected, use jaw thrust during bag—mask ventilation.

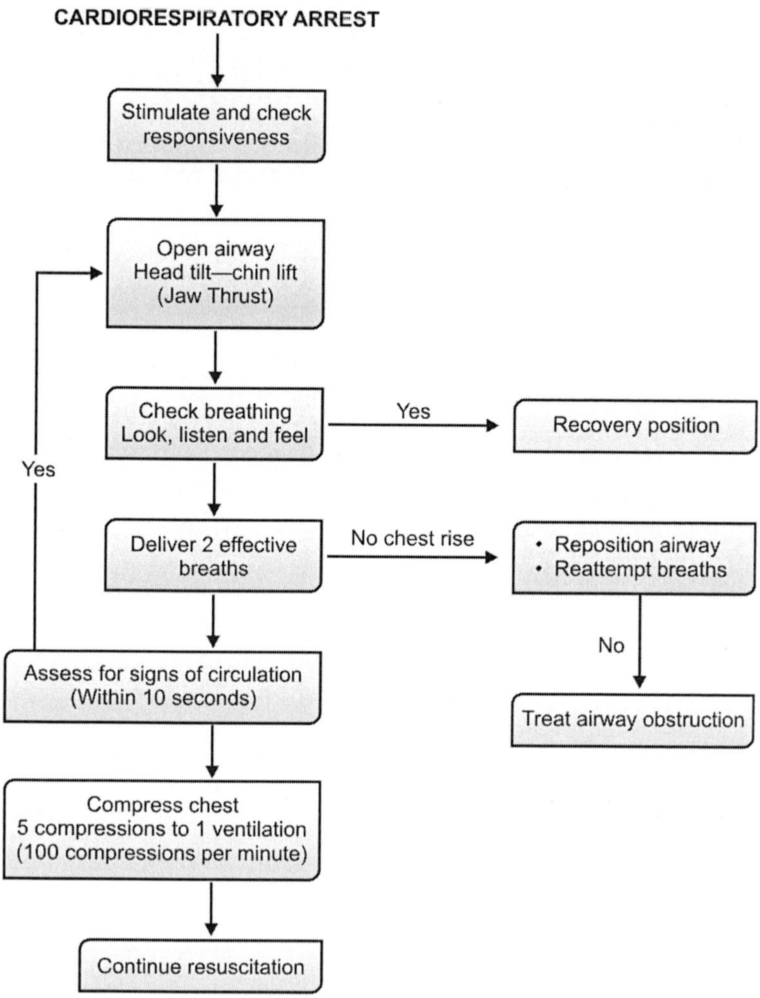

- When FBAO is suspected in unresponsive child use the tongue —jaw lift
- 2-5 rescue breaths can be given to ensure that at least 2 effective ventilations are provided.
- Volume of each rescue breath should be sufficient to rise the chest visibly. If air enters freely and chest rises the airway is clear.
- Cricoid pressure will decrease gastric inflation in unconscious or unresponsive child during bag and mask ventilation.
- If there is no chest rise even after repositioning and reopening airway, treat the victim for presumed FBAO.
- Resuscitation bags used for ventilation of full-term newborns, infants and children should have a minimum volume of 450-500 ml. Regardless of the size of the resuscitator used, the rescuer should use only the force and tidal volume necessary to cause the chest to rise.
- Avoid excessive tidal volume in small airway obstruction (Causes air trapping, baro trauma and reduced cardiac output) and head injury.
- Use bracheal pulse in infant and carotid pulse in child for pulse check.
- Pulse check should take no more than 10 seconds.
- Profound bradycardia with poor perfusion is an indication for chest compression.
- In newborn chest should be compressed to one third its depth. For the infant or child depth of compression is one third to one half of the depth of chest.
- Compress lower half of sternum. Avoid compressing the xiphoid process.
- Chest compressions should produce palpable pulses in a central artery.
- The compression (downward) and relaxation (upward) time during each compression cycle should be approximately equal. Do not lift fingers from sternum during a cycle or in between cycles.

2

Pediatric Advanced Life Support Guidelines

The Pediatric Advanced Life Support Guidelines are shown in following flowchart.

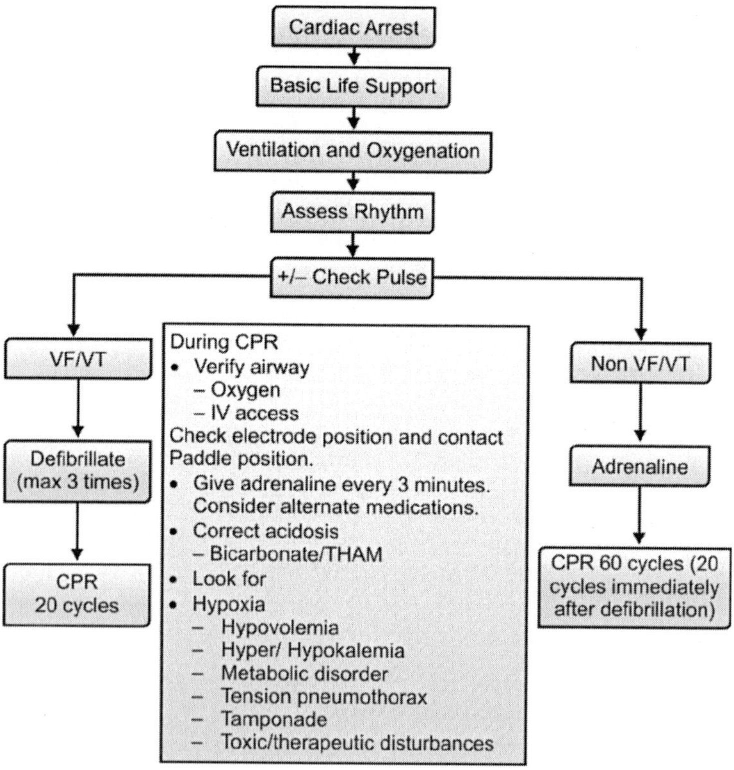

3

Automated External Defibrillators

- AED evaluates the victim's ECG to determine if a "shockable" rhythm is present, charges to an appropriate dose and when activated delivers a shock.
- Experience with AEDs in children is very limited. Used in children older than 8 years.
- Defibrillation with AEDs in children younger than 8 years currently carries an Indeterminate class of recommendation (PALS).
- BLS remains the initial treatment of choice for victims of all ages in cardiac arrest associated with asphyxia.
- After 3 shocks or whenever the AED indicates "no shock indicated," check airway, breathing and circulation and provide CPR as indicated for 1 minute, then reanalyze rhythm and provide more shocks if needed.

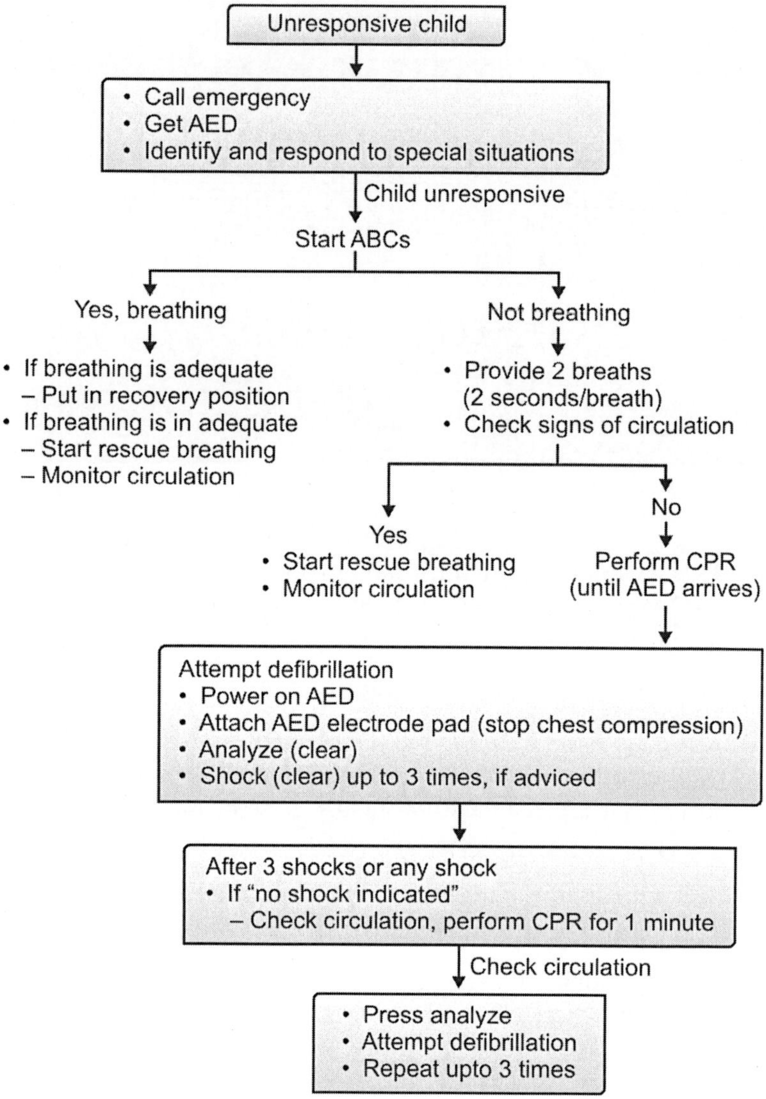
Unresponsive child
• Call emergency
• Get AED
• Identify and respond to special situations
Child unresponsive
Start ABCs
Yes, breathing
• If breathing is adequate
– Put in recovery position
• If breathing is in adequate
– Start rescue breathing
– Monitor circulation
Not breathing
• Provide 2 breaths (2 seconds/breath)
• Check signs of circulation
Yes
• Start rescue breathing
• Monitor circulation
No
Perform CPR (until AED arrives)
Attempt defibrillation
• Power on AED
• Attach AED electrode pad (stop chest compression)
• Analyze (clear)
• Shock (clear) up to 3 times, if adviced
After 3 shocks or any shock
• If "no shock indicated"
– Check circulation, perform CPR for 1 minute
Check circulation
• Press analyze
• Attempt defibrillation
• Repeat upto 3 times

4

Bradycardia Algorithm

- Clinically significant bradycardia is defined as heart rate less than 60 bpm associated with poor systemic perfusion.
- Bradyarrhythmias are the most common pre arrest rhythm in the pediatric patient and are often associated with hypoxemia, hypotension and acidosis.
- Most clinically significant bradycardia are caused by hypoxemia, so immediate support of airway, ventilation and oxygenation is warranted.
- The action of catecholamines may be reduced by acidosis and hypoxemia making support of oxygenation and ventilation essential for the optimal action of the drugs used.
- Continuous epinephrine or dopamine infusion may be useful.
- If bradycardia is known or strongly suspected to be caused by increased vagal tone or primary AV block, administer atropine preferentially after establishment of oxygenation and ventilation.
- If IV access is not readily available, atropine may be administered tracheally. The absorption may be unreliable and a larger dose may be required.
- Small doses of atropine may produce paradoxical bradycardia, hence minimum dose of 0.1 mg is recommended.
- Pacing is not useful in children with asystole or with bradycardia secondary to a postarrest hypoxic myocardial insult or respiratory failure.

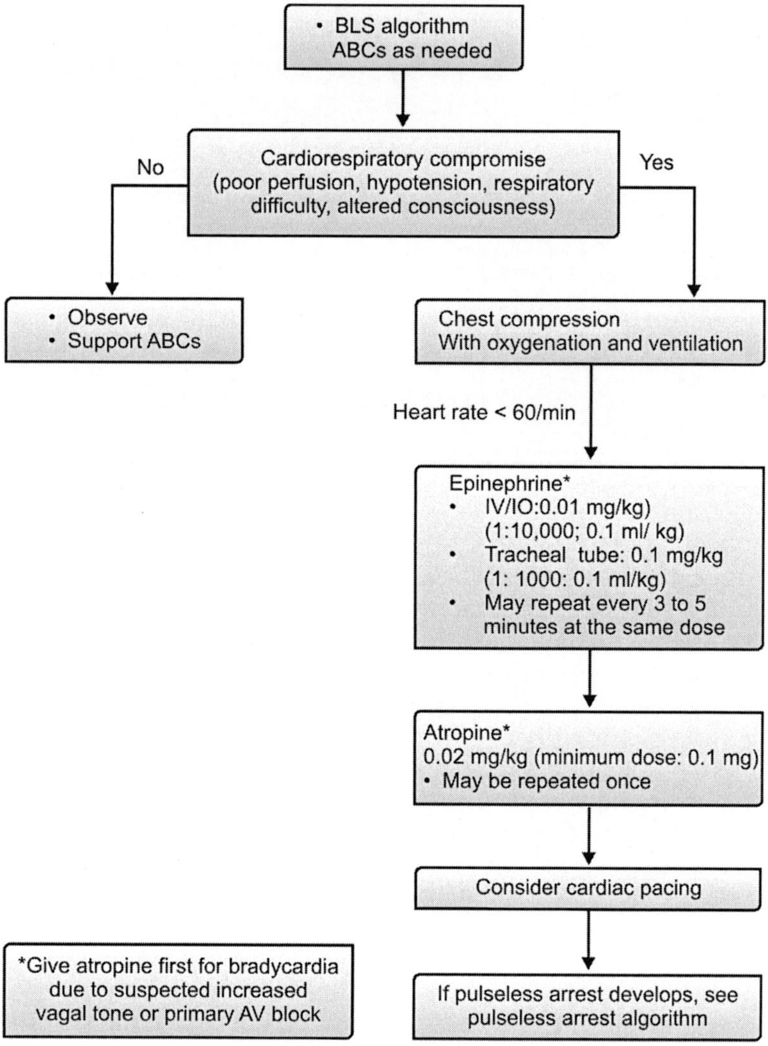
• BLS algorithm
ABCs as needed
Cardiorespiratory compromise
(poor perfusion, hypotension, respiratory difficulty, altered consciousness)
No
Yes
• Observe
• Support ABCs
Chest compression
With oxygenation and ventilation
Heart rate < 60/min
Epinephrine*
• IV/IO:0.01 mg/kg)
(1:10,000; 0.1 ml/ kg)
• Tracheal tube: 0.1 mg/kg
(1: 1000: 0.1 ml/kg)
• May repeat every 3 to 5 minutes at the same dose
Atropine*
0.02 mg/kg (minimum dose: 0.1 mg)
• May be repeated once
Consider cardiac pacing
If pulseless arrest develops, see pulseless arrest algorithm
*Give atropine first for bradycardia due to suspected increased vagal tone or primary AV block

5

Pulseless Arrest

- Pulseless arrest is also called collapse rhythm. Patient with collapse rhythm have no signs of perfusion.
- VF, pulseless VT, asystole and pulseless electrical activity (PEA) are collapse rhythms.
- Most common arrest rhythm in pediatric age group is asystole.
- It is important to identifying nonasystolic causes of arrest, because in many studies survival rate from VF/pulseless VT arrest is higher than survival rate from asystole.
- If collapse is sudden, with known risk factors for cardiac disease, VF/pulseless VT is more likely. Prepare for immediate rhythm analysis and defibrillation.
- If arrest occurs with risk factors for hypoxia or ischemia preceding the arrest, asystole is more likely. Emphasis should be on early support of airway and oxygenation.
- A systole is associated with absent electrical activity represented by a flat line on ECG. Confirm clinically the absence of signs of circulation, because a "flat line" ECG can be caused by a loose ECG lead.
- If possible confirm asystole in more than one ECG lead to identify very fine VF.
- Asystole is most common rhythm observed in infants and children presenting with out-of-hospital cardiac arrest. It is

almost always associated with hypoxia and ischemia. Prognosis for intact neurological survival is poor.

- High dose epinephrine may be considered for special circumstances like anaphylaxis, known α and β blocker

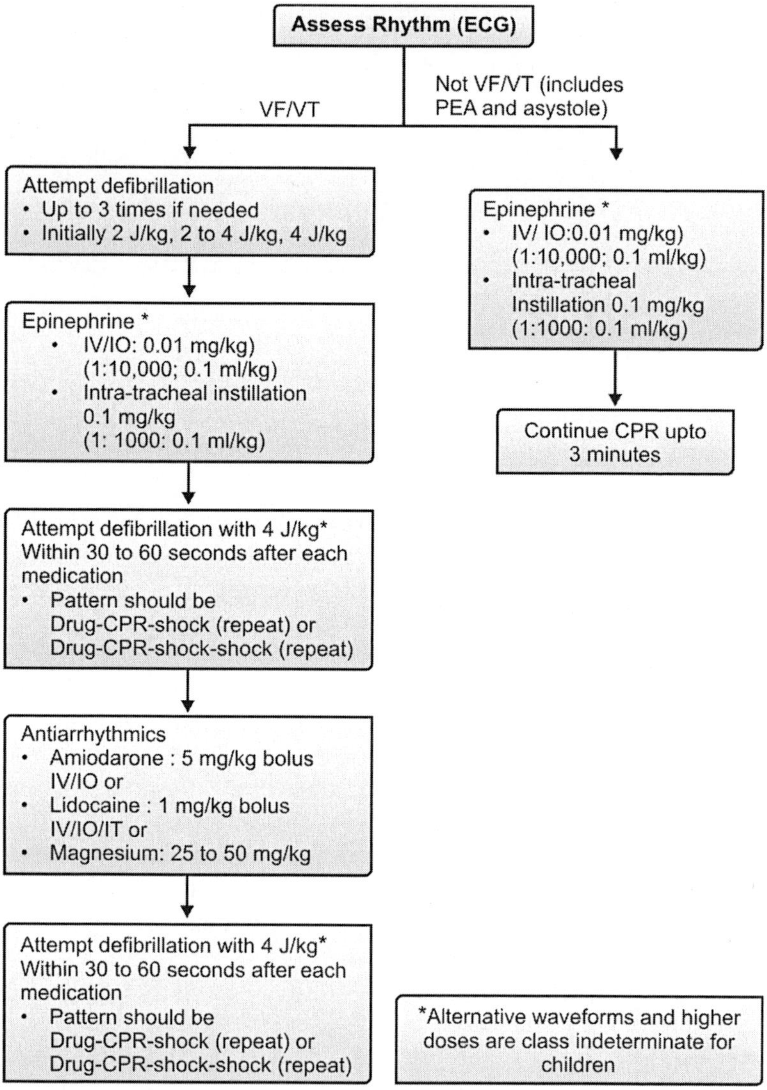

overdose, child with severe sepsis already receiving high dose vasopressor.

- Pulseless electrical activity (PEA) is electrical activity other than VF or VT that does not produce a palpable arterial pulse. PEA may be reversible if it is identified early and treated appropriately.
- Aggressively treat any patient with PEA. These patients need volume expansion, nor epinephrine, dopamine or some combination of the therapies.

6

Tachycardia Algorithm

- In a child with rapid heart rate, initial evaluation should consider
  - Whether child has a pulse and signs of circulation. If child has rapid pulse, continue with tachycardia algorithm. If patient has no pulse, initiate the pulseless arrest algorithm.
  - Is perfusion adequate or poor? If perfusion is adequate, proceed to tachycardia with adequate perfusion algorithm. If there is poor perfusion, proceed immediately to algorithm for tachycardia with poor perfusion.

To correct sinus tachycardia (ST), treat the underlying cause. Do not attempt to decrease heart rate by pharmalogical or electrical interventions.

The child with ST usually has a history consistent with possible causes of tachycardia whereas child with supraventricular tachycardia (SVT) has history incompatible with tachycardia.

ST and SVT can be differentiated with ECG characteristics:

- Heart rates above 180 bpm are more likely to be SVT in infants and older children. Whereas newborns can often have ST at rates greater than 200 bpm.
- SVT is initially well-tolerated in infants and older children. Cardiac output is significantly impaired after prolonged episode.

- Hemodynamic instability or shock is not helpful for differentiating SVT and VT.
- Synchronized electrical cardioversion is recommended to treat SVT with poor perfusion, although adenosine may be administered if IV or IO access is immediately available. Do

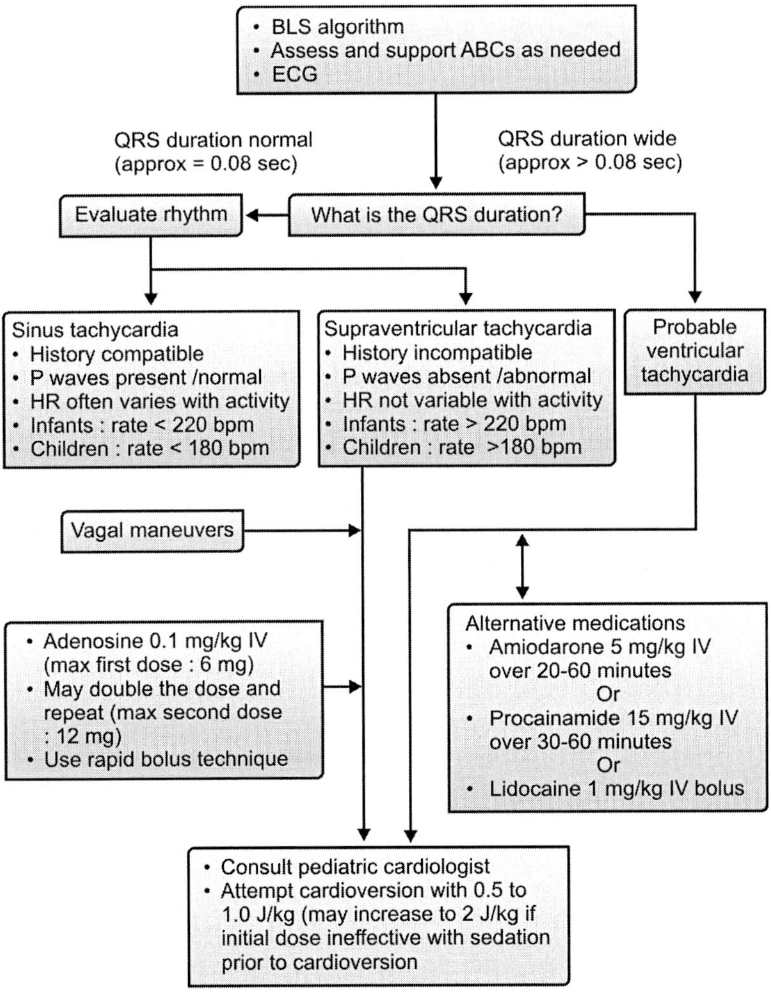

Note :

- SVT and VT with poor perfusion immediate cardioversion with 0.5 to 1.0 J/kg
- Do not administer amiodarone and procainamide together.

not delay cardioversion to establish vascular access. During preparation for electrical or chemical cardioversion, a brief trial of vagal maneuvers may be tried, without delaying the cardioversion.

- Vagal maneuvers—try applying ice water to face of the infant without obstructing ventilation. Ask child to blow through an obstructed straw to induce vagal response. Do not apply ocular pressure or provide carotid massage.
- Provide sedation with analgesia, if it will not delay cardioversion.
- SVT with adequate perfusion is more common and less emergent. Adenosine is the drug of choice.
- Common cause of adenosine failing to convert SVT is that the drug is administered too slowly. Use rapid flush technique.
- VT is uncommon in pediatric age group. Ventricular rate in VT may vary from near normal to more than 200 bpm. VT may deteriorate into pulseless VT or VF.
- Most children who develop VT have underlying structural heart disease, prolonged QT syndrome or myocarditis. Previously undiagnosed wide—QRS tachycardia in an infant or child should be treated as VT unless proved otherwise.
- Ventricular tachycardia (VT)—after third shock, give epinephrine, continue CPR for 30 to 60 seconds to allow epinephrine to circulate. Attempt defibrillation with 4 J/kg. Pattern of action should be drug –CPR- shock.
- Defibrillate with three shocks in quick succession. Between shocks, the paddles should remain on the chest while rhythm is quickly reassessed. Perform pulse check only after the third shock.
- Epinephrine in high dose was considered mainstay of therapy for shock resistant pulseless VT/VF. Recent studies have shown that epinephrine in standard dose was better than high-dose epinephrine. Standard dose should be used for the initial and subsequent doses.
- Do not miss "fine VF." If there is any doubt defibrillation should be attempted.

7

Rapid Sequence Intubation

- Sedation and paralysis are recommended for intubation except in newborns, unconscious and patients with cardiorespiratory arrest.
- Endotracheal tube (ETT) size: (age + 16) ÷ 4 = internal diameter of ETT (mm)
- Have one ETT 0.5 mm smaller and one ETT 0.5 mm larger than estimated size.
- An uncuffed ETT should be used in child < 8 years old. Depth of insertion (in cms; at teeth and lips) is about 3 times the ETT size.
- Laryngoscope; a straight blade can be used in all patients.
- Attach bag and mask to 100% oxygen.
- ETT stylets should not exceed beyond distal end of ETT.
- Intubation attempts should not exceed 30 seconds.
- Varify ETT placement by chest wall movement, auscultation, capnometer, Presence of water vapors in tube, improvement in saturation or chest radiograph.
- Remove cricoid pressure only after verifying ETT placement.
- Preoxygenation with 100% oxygen allows for a period of apnea without desaturation during the procedure. Normal 10 kg child will desaturate to below 90% in approximately 3.5 minutes of apnea and a critically ill child with pulmonary disease will desaturate more quickly.

RAPID SEQUENCE INTUBATION MEDICATIONS

Drug	*Dose (IV) mg/kg*	*Comments*
Adjuncts (first)		
Atropine	0.01-0.02 min:0.1 mg max:1 mg	Vagolytic, prevents bradycardia and reduces oral secretions, may increase HR.
Lidocaine	1-2	Optional anestheic blunts ICP spike, cough reflex and CV effects of intubation controls ventricular arrhythmias.
Sedative – Hypnotic (second)		
Thiopental	1-7	May cause myocardial depression use low dose (1-2) in hypovolemia. Causes broncho and laryngospasm. C/I in status asthmaticus.
Ketamine	1-3	May increase ICP, BP, HR causes bronchodilation give with atropine.
Midazolam	0.05-0.1	May cause decreased BP and HR, respiratory depression; amnestic properties
Fentanyl	1-5 mcg/kg	Least hemodynamic effects of all opiates. chest wall rigidity with high-dose or rapid administration. Action reversible with naloxone.
Paralytics (Third)		
Vecuronium	0.1- 0.2	Onset 70-120 sec. Duration 30-90 min. Minimal effect on BP and HR. May reverse in 30-45 minutes with atropine and neostigmine
Succinylcholine	1-2	Onset 30-60 sec; duration 30-10 min; increases ICP, reversible. C/I in burns, massive trauma, neuromuscular disease.

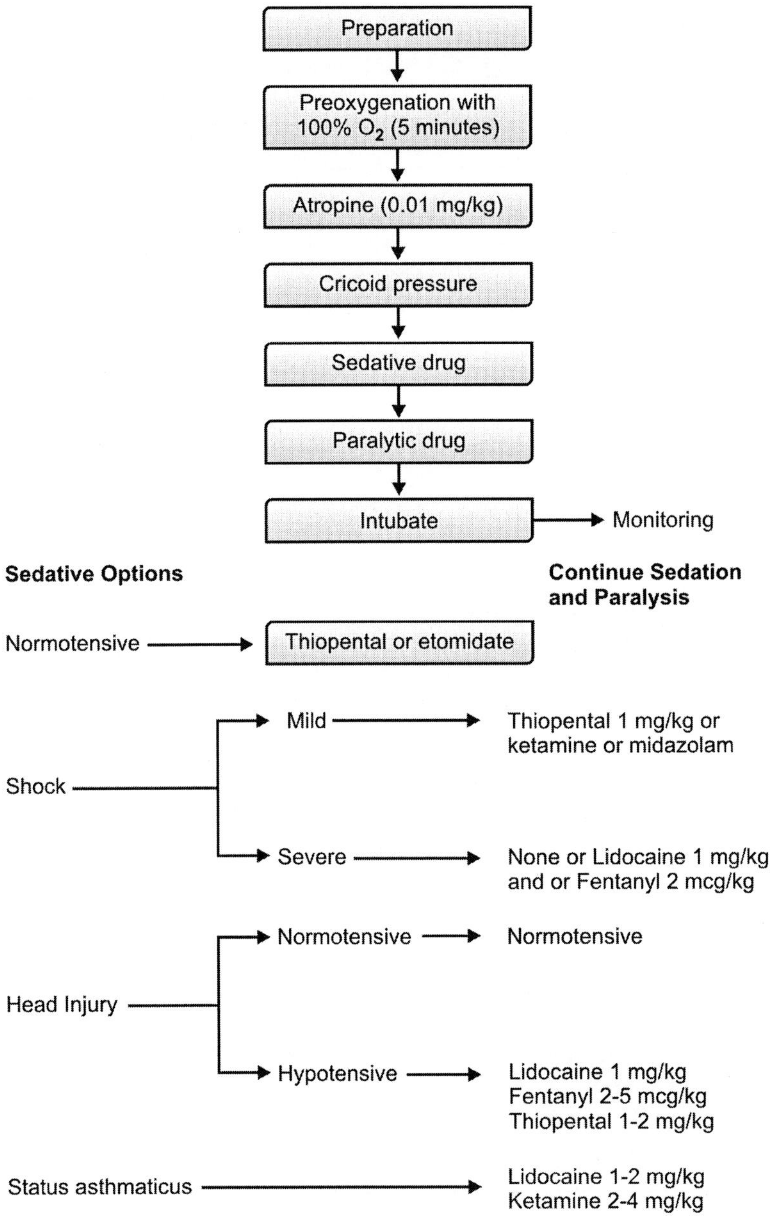
Preparation
Preoxygenation with 100% O_2 (5 minutes)
Atropine (0.01 mg/kg)
Cricoid pressure
Sedative drug
Paralytic drug
Intubate
Monitoring
Sedative Options
Continue Sedation and Paralysis
Normotensive
Thiopental or etomidate
Shock
Mild
Thiopental 1 mg/kg or ketamine or midazolam
Severe
None or Lidocaine 1 mg/kg and or Fentanyl 2 mcg/kg
Head Injury
Normotensive
Normotensive
Hypotensive
Lidocaine 1 mg/kg
Fentanyl 2-5 mcg/kg
Thiopental 1-2 mg/kg
Status asthmaticus
Lidocaine 1-2 mg/kg
Ketamine 2-4 mg/kg

8

Anaphylaxis

- Most common symptoms of anaphylaxis are urticaria and angio-edema. 90% patients with anaphylaxis experience at least one of these two symptoms. However, not all patients will have these symptoms and may present only with cardiovascular collapse (anaphylactic shock).
- Atopic individuals have increased risk of experiencing an anaphylactic reaction. Atopic individuals with poorly controlled asthma are at increased risk of severe anaphylactic reaction and death.
- Patients presenting with critical symptoms as stridor or severe hypotension, epinephrine should be given IM immediately and switched to IV dosing as vascular access is obtained.
- Some studies have indicated that IM route is better than SC in anaphylaxis. Give IM injection at lateral aspect of thigh.
- Critical patients require aggressive fluid resuscitation due to massive fluid shifts.
- Nebulized salbutamol—quick estimation of required dose; 2.5 mg for < 30 kg, 5 mg for > 30 kg.
- Corticosteriods are given to prevent late phase of allergic response. Give methylprednisalone 2 mg/kg/d divided every 6 hourly or prednisalone 2 mg/kg PO.OD.
  Observe for 6-24 hours for late phase symptoms.

Additional pharmacological therapy plays very important role in the management of anaphylaxis. H_1 and H_2 blockers should be given to all patients with anaphylaxis.

Check ABCs – initial assessment.

Establish airway, 100% O_2 support respiration.

Epinephrine 0.01ml/kg(1:1000), SC/IM.

- Check circulation.
- Put patients head at 30° angle below feet.
- Give NS 20 ml/kg IV over 5–10 minute repeat bolus as necessary.
- Epinephrine 0.1 ml/kg (1:10,000) may be given IV over 2-5 min.

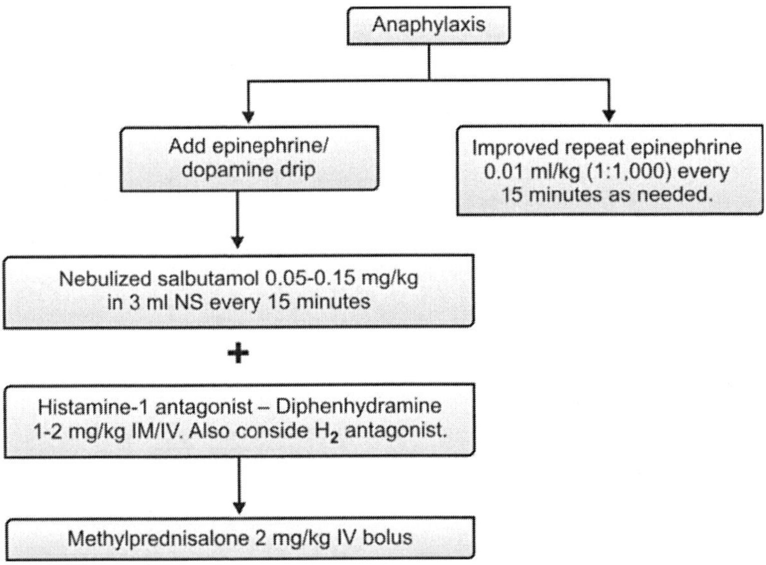

9

Congestive Cardiac Failure

Congestive Cardiac Failure (CCF) is shown as given below:

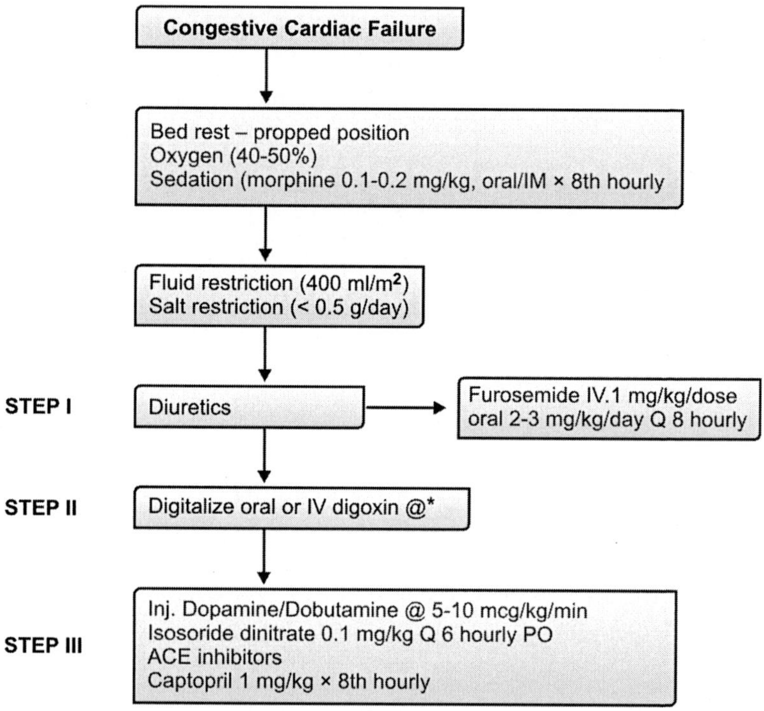

* @ Digitalizing dose for premature infants : 0.04 mg/kg/day

Full-term neonates	: 0.06 mg/kg/day
Children < 2 years of age	: 0.06-0.08 mg/kg/day
Children > 2 years of age	: 0.04 mg/kg/day

- Parental dose is 2/3rd of this amount.
- One half of digitalizing dose is given stat followed by 1/4th after 8 hours and 1/4th after 16 hours.
- The daily maintenance digoxin is about 1/4th of initial digitalizing dose.

Caution: Hyokalemia, hypercalcemia, hypomagnesemia

Failure to Respond

- Review of medication and dosage
- Review of contributory factors
  - Hypertension
  - Low blood sugar
  - Dyselectolytemia
  - Acidosis, Anemia
  - Fluid overload
  - Myocarditis/cardiomyopathy

Other Drugs Used

Amrinone/Milrinone

Loading dose of 0.75 mg/kg IV followed by intravenous infusion of 5-10 mg/kg/min

Amiodarone

Useful in atrial fibrillation and ventricular tachycardia.

10

Cyanotic Spell

Cyanotic Spell is defined as under:

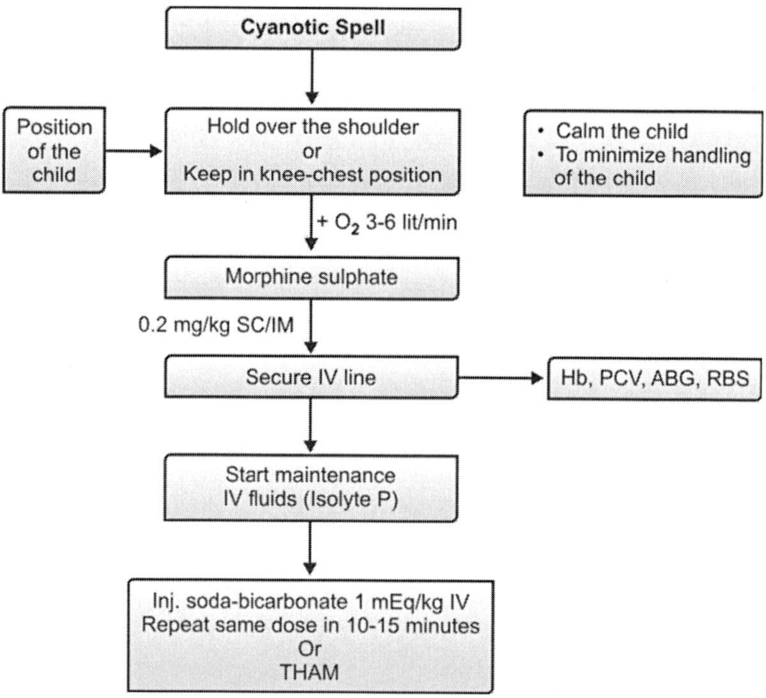

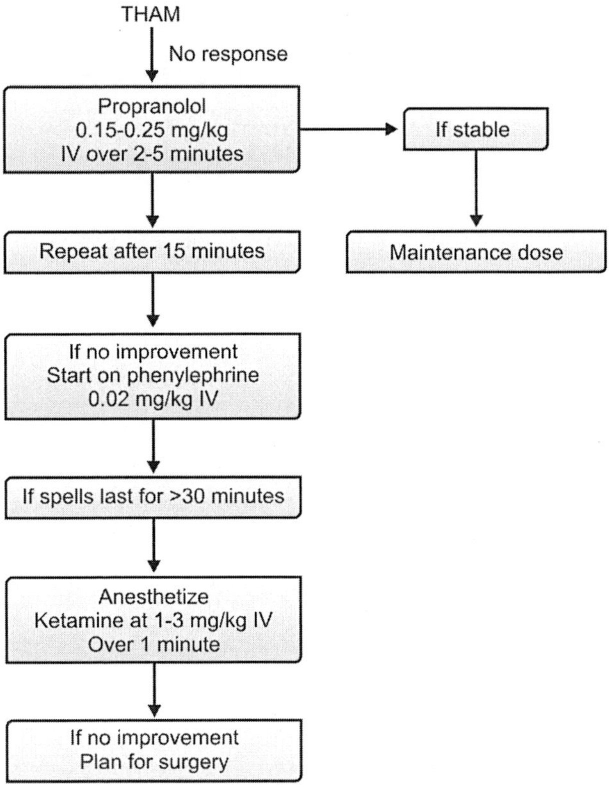

Note : IV fluids to be started even when well-hydrated as polycythemia predisposes to dehydration.

11

Shock

- Expansion of circulating blood volume is a critical component of treatment of circulatory shock.
- Volume expansion is best achieved with isotonic crystalloid solutions. They are readily available, inexpensive and do not produce sensitivity reactions.
- Only 1/4th of crystalloid solution remains in intravascular compartment. As a result a large quantity (4-5 times the deficit) should be given. Rapid infusion of this quantity is well-tolerated by healthy young patient.
- Blood products should be administered for replacement of blood loss or correction of coagulopathies. Blood is recommended for fluid replacement of volume loss in trauma victims with poor perfusion despite administration of 2-3 boluses of crystalloid solution. Transfuse blood if hematocrit is less than 30%.
- Volume therapy is indicated when a child demonstrates early signs of shock. Prompt and effective treatment of compensated shock may prevent development of decompensated shock and morbidity and mortality associated with it.
- For shock resuscitation the PALS guidelines recommend administration of fluid boluses over 5-20 minutes.
- In severe hypovolemia give 20 ml/kg bolus rapidly over 5-10 minutes. If child has less severe signs of shock or there is possibility of myocardial impairment (calcium channel blocker

or β-adrenergic blocker poisoning) administer bolus over 10-20 minutes.

- Dopamine infusion rate greater than 20 mcg/kg/min may produce vasoconstricitve effects without further inotropic effect. If additional inotropic effect is needed epinephrine or dobutamine may be preferable. If further vasopressor support is needed to maintain blood pressure, epinephrine or norepinephrine is generally preferred.
- Dopamine infusion should be given through a secure, large bore peripheral venous catheter. Extravasation can result in local ischemia and tissue necrosis.
- Dopamine and other catecholamines should not be mixed with sodium bicarbonate.
- There is wide interpatient variability in pharmacokinetics of dopamine and hemodynamic responses to it. Therefore titrate infusion rate to desired clinical response. Vasopressors should be titrated to the desired effect. Tachyarrhythmia can be dose limiting and may require changing therapy.
- Dobutamine may be less effective than epinephrine in septic shock particularly, if hypotension is present, because dobutamine may increase existing systemic vasodilation.
- Dobutamine is an effective agent for treatment of poor perfusion despite adequate intravascular volume.
- Indications for epinephrine infusion are poor perfusion or hypotension in the patient with adequate intravascular volume and stable rhythm. It is also indicated in hemodynamically significant bradycardia, pulseless arrest.
- Epinephrine acts directly on adrenergic receptor unlike dopamine, which acts through release of stored nor epinephrine. Epinephrine may be preferable to dopamine for the patient with depleted norepinephrine stores such as chronic congestive cardiac failure.
- Inodilators (milrinone) may be administered to augment cardiac output and reduce systemic vascular resistance.
- Hypoglycemia is common in septic shock especially in infants. In addition critically ill and septic children often have low ionized calcium. Hypoglycemia and hypocalcemia can contribute to cardiac dysfunction. Both conditions should be identified and treated.
- No clear consensus for steroid use in pediatric shock. Use in children with underlying hypothalamic or pituitary

dysfunction, prolonged steroid use or in children with severe septic shock with purpura.

Therapeutic Endpoints in the Treatment of Shock

- CFT < 2 sec. Normal pulses with no difference between peripheral and central pulses.
- Urine output >1 ml/kg/hr.
- Normal mental status.
- Decreased lactate and base excess.

Airway	: Maintain airway
Breathing	: 100% oxygen Consider early intubation
Circulation	: Establish venous access/Intraosseous access Rapid infusion of 20 ml/kg fluid RL/NS Upto 60 ml/kg over 15 min. Correct hypoglycemia (25% dextrose 2-4 ml/kg. bolus) Correct hypocalcemia (2 ml/kg of 10% calcium gluconate)

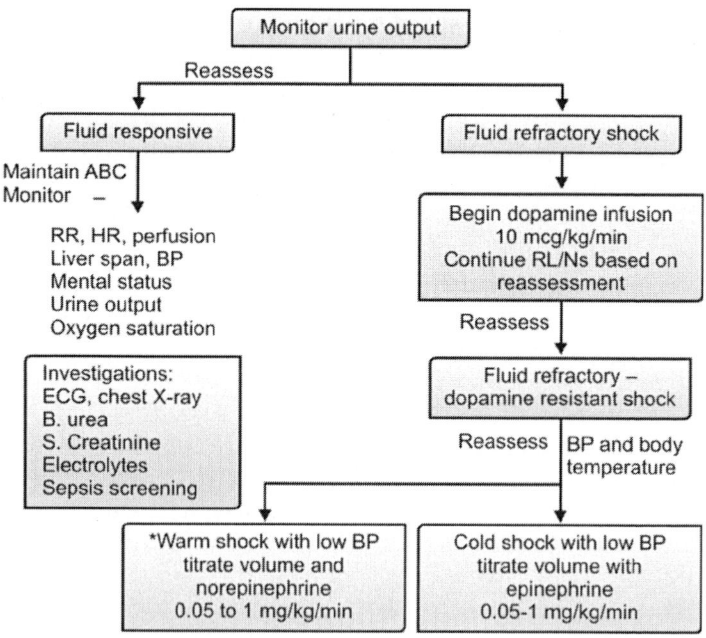

Catecholamine Resistant Shock

At risk of adrenal insufficiency
Hydrocortisone 50 mg/kg. bolus
Followed by infusion of
50 mg/kg/24 hours

No risk of adrenal insufficiency
Do not give Inj. hydrocortisone

Note:

Stop Bolus and start dopamine if

- Work of breathing increases
- Onset of new rales
- Gallop rhythm
- Liver span increasing

Indications for intubation

- Airway unstable/gasping
- Work of breathing increasing due to cardiogenic shock on arrival
- Hypoventilation or respiratory failure GCS £ 8
- Depending on central venous pressure

CVP > 15 mm

Repeated isotonic crystalloid
Or colloids (5-10 ml/kg)

Reassess

Continue fluid water
CVP monitoring
Consider alternate

Cold shock – CFT > 2 secs
Mottled cool extremities

Warm shock. Flash capillary refill
Bounding peripheral pulses.

HgCVP 10-15 mm

Inotrope

HgCVP < 10 mm Hg

Consider
– Diuretics
– Dialysis

12

Burns

- Use burn assessment chart to map areas of second and third degree burns.
- Body surface area (BSA) of burns is based only on percentage of second degree burns.
- The extent and severity of burn injury can change in the first day. Reassess the child frequently and do not prognosticate depending on initial assessment.
- Consider intubation when there is evidence of inhalation injury, for pulmonary toilet, for burns greater than 25% BSA.
- Inhalation is present in 30% of victims of major flame burns, and should be considered when there is evidence of fire in enclosed space, charring of lips, hoarseness, cough or wheezing. Inhalation injury increases mortality.
- Mortality of scald/contact burns is similar to that in flame burns when total BSA involved is equivalent.
- All patients with large burns and/closed space burns should be assumed to have carbon monoxide poisoning until examination and evaluation of blood carboxyhemoglobin is undertaken. Humidified 100% O_2 oxygen should be administered during initial assessment.
- Increasing tachypnea may be due to acute asphyxia and CO toxicity, upper airway obstruction secondary to edema, and overwhelming lung parenchymal damage.

- Start fluid resuscitation in infants with burns greater than 10% of BSA or children with burns greater than 15% BSA or children with evidence of smoke inhalation.
- Consider central venous access for burns > 25% BSA.
- Cooling decreases the severity of burns, if administered within 30 minutes of injury. It also helps to relieve pain. If burn is less than 10% of BSA, apply clean towels soaked in cold water to reduce burn progression. If burns are more than 10% of BSA, apply clean, dry towels to burn to avoid hypothermia.
- IV analgesia is often necessary to treat pain. Do not attribute anxiety or restlessness to pain until adequate perfusion, oxygenation and ventilation are established.
- Consider adding colloids after 18-24 hours to maintain serum albumin > 2g/dl.
- Withhold potassium for first 48 hours. Monitor urine electrolytes and replace urine losses accordingly.

First Aid at the Scene of Accident

- Burns <10% of BSA apply wet towel to prevent burn progression
- >10% BSA—apply dry towel to avoid heat loss
- Chemical burns—wash with water for 20 minutes or neutralize it.

Primary Survey

- Maintain airway—intubation if needed + mechanical ventilation
- Breathing—start with high flow oxygen
- Circulation—start IV line (atleast – 2)
- Start IV fluids ringer lactate 20 ml/kg, if child is in shock
- Assessment of extent of burns
- Blood for Hb, PCV, urea, creatinine, electrolytes
- Sedation, Take weight it patient is stable.

Secondary Survey

- Assessment of area and depth of burnt surface. Start fluid therapy, correct initial shock with ringer lactate (20 ml/kg).

First 24 hours (Parkland's formula)

Ringer Lactate (4 ml/kg/% of burn) Therapy

- 1/2 the amount in 1st 8 hours
- 1/2 in next 16 hours.

Second 24 hours

- 5% dextrose with N/4 or N/2 saline maintenance fluids
- Plasma or albumin administration
- Continue fluids till BP and CVP above normal.

Other Supportive Management

- Keep child NPO in case of severe burns
- Decompression of stomach with nasogastric tube
- ORS, breast feeds if < 5% burns
- Oxygen therapy
- Sedation with parentral pethidine or diazepam
- Monitor vital parameters
- Monitor urinary output
- Nutrition – enteral feeds by 3 days
- Antibiotics
- Wounds care.

Note:

PCV > 24% – Packed cells

*low protein levels – Albumin colloid formula

30-50% BSA	0.3 ml/kg
50-70% BSA	0.4 ml/kg
70-100% BSA	0.5 ml/kg

- 5% dextrose to be added to RL in children < 5 years old
- Change fluids according to electrolyte/acid-base values.

13

Near Drowning

INTRODUCTION

- Heimlich maneuver has not been shown to be effective in removing aspirated water.
- Initiate rescue breathing immediately, even while the patient is still in the water, if necessary and feasible. Chest compressions are not effective in the water and waste valuable time.
- Remove debris in oropharynx by Finger-sweep technique.
- The most critical role in management is prompt correction of hypoxemia and acidosis.
- Higher pressure required for ventilation due to poor compliance of lungs (caused by pulmonary edema).
- Consider intubation and mechanical ventilation in any patient with poor respiratory effort, altered sensorium, severe hypoxemia, severe acidosis, or significant respiratory distress
- Hypothermia may also exist and exacerbate bradycardia, acidosis, and hypoxia.
- Patients with severe hypothermia may appear dead because of profound bradycardia and vasoconstriction. Resuscitation should continue while aggressive attempts are made to restore normal body temperature.

- Consider potential spinal injuries, especially in diving accidents. Associated injuries must be considered, as in any other form of accidental injury.
- Ventricular dysarrhythmias, bradycardia and asystole are often due to hypoxemia rather than electrolyte imbalance.
- Acidosis is corrected after correction of volume depletion and oxygenation. Sodium bicarbonate can be used for severe acidosis but only after adequate ventilation has been established.
- Intravascular volume depletion is common regardless of type of water aspirated.
- Supplemental oxygen 100% should be administered as soon as available.
- Degree of hypoxia may be difficult to determine on clinical observation, hence monitoring is required.

Complications

Immediate complications are secondary to hypoxia and acidosis. The immediate threats are the effects on the CNS and cardiovascular systems. CNS effects depend on the severity and duration of hypoxia. Posthypoxic cerebral hypoperfusion may occur. Long-term effects of cerebral hypoxia, including vegetative survival, are the most devastating. Hypoxia and acidosis may lead to cardiac dysrhythmias, including ventricular fibrillation and asystole. Myocardial damage may lead to cardiogenic shock. Capillary leak and neurologic injury can predispose submersion victims to hypovolemia and hypotension. Aspiration of fresh or salt water alters the function of surfactant, causing injury to the alveoli and pulmonary capillaries.

Near drowning patients may develop pneumonia, although it is less common than chemical pneumonitis, especially if the submersion occurs in a chlorinated pool or in a bucket containing a cleaning product.

- *Secure an airway*:
  - Intubation and ventilation with PEEP in case of respiratory distress
  - Glasgow's score < 8 or deteriorating
  - Severe myocardial dysfunction

- Breathing : Aim to maintain $SPO_2 > 90\%$
- Empty the stomach using Ryle's tube
- **IV fluids**

  Fresh water: Normal maintenance fluid (NS)

  Sea water: If perfusion poor
  - 20 ml/kg isotonic normal saline bolus up to 2 boluses
  - Plasma or plasma substitutes are preferred
  - Maintenance fluid

Investigations
Chest X-ray
ABG
Hb, S. Protein
S. Electrolytes
Urine analysis
Urine fibrin degradation products

- Maintain temperature at 36-36.5°C
  - Cover with blankets
  - IV fluids warmed to 40-42°C
- Corrections of acidosis

  1-2 ml/kg IV soda bicarbonate
- *Treat convulsions*:
  - Phenobarbitone 15-20 mg/kg loading dose IV, maintenance with 5-8 mg/kg/day or
  - Diazepam 0.2- 0.3 mg/kg IV or
  - Phenytoin loading dose 15-20 mg/kg IV infusion rare 1 mg/kg/min, maintenance with 5-8 mg/kg/day
  - Q 12H
- *Treat raised intracranial tension*
  - Raise head end of bed
  - Mannitol 20% 5 ml/kg stat

    2 ml/kg Q 6 H × 2 days
  - Hyperventilation if on ventilator
- In pulmonary edema
  - 5% glucose normal saline maintance
  - Furosemide 1-2 mg/kg/day IV
  - Positive pressure ventilation.
- In congestive cardiac failure
  - Fluid restriction
  - Oxygen inhalation

  - Furosemide 1-2 mg/kg/day IV
  - Digoxin
- *IV antibiotics*: Prophylactic antibiotics have no role in management. Indicated in
  - Established infections only
  - Persistent fever
  - Drowning in contaminated fluid.

14

Oxygen Therapy

INTRODUCTION

- Successful treatment of tissue hypoxia requires early recognition. Clinical features of hypoxia are nonspecific and include dyspnea, altered mental status.
- Pulse oxymetry and PaO_2 are principal indicators of initiating, monitoring and adjusting oxygen therapy. However, SPO_2 and PaO_2 can be normal when tissue hypoxia is caused by low output cardiac states, anemia and failure of tissues to utilize oxygen.
- Oxygen delivery system can be low- flow system or high-flow system. Low-flow system provides an FiO_2 that varies with the patient's inspiratory flow. High-flow system provides a specific FiO_2 at flows that meet or exceed patient's inspiratory flow requirements.
- Maximum flow accepted through nasal cannula is 2L/min and humidification of oxygen is not necessary as oxygen flows from cannula to nasopharynx, which acts as reservoir.
- Improper size cannula or high-rate of gas flow can lead to inadvertent CPAP administration.
- Oxygen mask—Reservoir effect is produced by internal capacity of mask. Rebreathing may result in accumulation of CO_2 if O_2

flow is inadequate. Aspiration of vomitus may be more likely when a mask is in place.

- Partial rebreathing masks contain a reservoir at the base of the mask. The reservoir receives fresh gas plus exhaled gas. This permits use of flow rates lower than those necessary for other devices.
- Non-rebreathing masks do not permit mixing of exhaled gases with fresh gas supply.
- Oxygen hood is a common method of administering oxygen to neonates and infants.Most hoods need a flow around 7L/min. FiO_2 achieved inside hood varies from 22 to 90% and depends on flow rate of oxygen, respiratory needs of baby, shape of the hoods and size of the side port openings.
- Maintain adequate heat and humidity inside the hood.
- 100% O_2 is indicated only for resuscitation and during transport of the child.
- Starting FiO_2 should be high in most cases (preferably 40-60%) using a high-flow device.
- Patient should be on high-flow system till cardiorespiratory status becomes stable.
- Minimum FiO_2 should be used to maintain the saturation of 92% and above.
- Avoid fluctuations in FiO_2.
- If 100% O_2 is required, it should not be denied for the fear of O_2 toxicity.

INDICATIONS

- Acute situations where O_2 saturation falls $< 90\%$ or $PaO_2 < 60$ mm Hg.
- Child with cardiac dysfunction (shock, cardiac failure) even if the patient has normal O_2 saturations.
- Any child with cyanosis or wheezing or stridor or RR > 50/minute (infants < 2 months with RR > 60/min) with intercostals recessions needs O_2.

OXYGEN DELIVERY DEVICES

Device	*Flow rate (L/min)*	*O_2 %*
Low Flow Systems (FiO_2 21- 60%)		
1. Nasal prongs/cannula	1	24
2. Simple facemask	4 -10	24-55%
3. Venturi mask	4 -10	25-60%
High Flow Systems (FiO_2 > 60%)		
1. Oxygen hood	10-15	80-90%
2. Partial rebreathing mask	10-12	60- 80%
3. Non-rebreathing mask	10-12	90-100%

Note:

- During CPR only 90-100% O_2 is advised, other O_2 delivery systems are used after stabilization.
- Nasal prongs/cannula are simple, well-tolerated and are the recommended devices to use in children.
- O_2 therapy should be monitored with pulse oximeter and ABG.
- Oxygen should not be stopped abruptly. It should be gradually tapered.
- Hyperbaric oxygen is used in carbon monoxide poisoning.

15

Croup

DO'S AND DON'TS IN SEVERE CROUP

Do's	*Dont's*
• Severe croup is a medical emergency. Examine and treat on a priority basis	• Do not panic
• Relieve the anxiety and try to comfort the baby	• Do not wake up the sleeping child with croup
• Administer humidified oxygen	• Do not move the baby out of mothers lap-avoid crying at all costs
• Try and arrange for a portable X-ray of neck	• Do not send the baby to the X-rays
• Arrange for a senior anesthetist and ENT surgeon	• Do not neglect the child till the X-rays are made available
• Secure an artificial airway expeditiously	• No venepuncture or intraveneous fluids till the airway has been established
• If pus is seen exuding from trachea, send for investigations and start antibiotics therapy.	• Do not wait for cultures before initiating treatment.

DOWNE'S SCORE FOR SIGNS OF UPPER AIRWAY OBSTRUCTION

		Score	
	0	*1*	*2*
• Stridor	None	Inspiratory	Inspiratory + Expiratory
• Cough	None	Hoarse cry	Barking
• Retractions + nasal flaring	None	Flaring + suprasternal, retractions	Flaring + suprasternal, subcostal, intercostals retractions
• Cyanosis	None	In air	In 40% oxygen
• Inspiratory breath sounds	Normal	Harsh with wheezing and/or rhonchi	Delayed
SCORES :	Up to 4 Mild	4-6 Moderate	> 6 Severe

MANAGEMENT

Mild Croup

- Minimal interference
- Continue oral feeds
- *Steroids*: Budesonide nebulization 2 mg in 4 ml NS

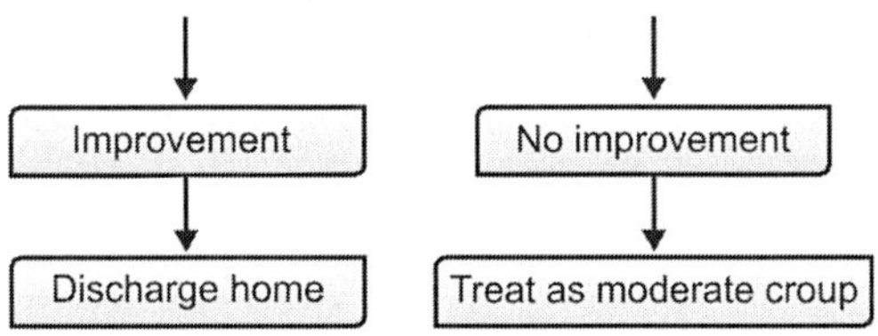

Moderate Croup

- NPO
- IV fluids
- Oxygen if $SPO_2 < 95\%$ (measured by pulse oximeter)
- Inhalation of nebulized adrenalin 1: 100
  1st dose : 1 ml in 3 ml NS
  2nd dose: 0.5 ml/kg can be repeated as required (max. 4 ml)
- *Steroids*
  - Dexamethasone 1 mg/kg IV stat followed by:
    1 mg /kg/day IV tid for 48-72 hours
    Budesonide nebulization 2 ml in 4 ml. NS single dose

Severe Croup

- Oxygen
- IV fluids
- Nebulized Adrenalin (dosage as above)
- Steroids: Combination (dosage above)
  - IV dexamethasone
  - Budesonide nebulization
- Immediate insertion of an artificial airway

To be done in ICU set-up:

- Endotracheal tube size should be one size smaller than recommended for age
- Intubation must be by an experienced person.
- Intubation is preferably done under deep halothane anesthesia.
- Humidification device must be attached.

16

Acute Asthma

- Assess HR, RR, and O_2 saturation, use of accessory muscles, alertness and color.
- Aerosol drug delivery is important aspect of asthma management. In ideal circumstances, only 10% medication reaches patient's airway. Moving the delivery device for short distance away can significantly affect the amount of medication delivered. All medications should be given through a snug fitting facemask.
- It is preferable to use oxygen rather than compressed air for nebulization in order to decrease the risk of desaturation caused by ventilation—perfusion mismatch. Flow rate should be 6-8 l/min to ensure proper granulation of nebulized substance.
- Drug delivery through spacer and mask is comparable to nebulizer. Given its shorter administration time and ease of use, spacer and mask should be considered in young children in place of nebulizer.
- β_2 agonists can be given with MDI to a co-operative child.
- β_2 agonists cause tachycardia and rarely tachyarrhytmias. Continuous nebulization can cause hypokalemia.
- Anticholinergics work as bronchodilators and also decrease airway secretions. They have little value when used alone. But

they are useful adjunctive with β-agonists in moderate exacerbations.

- Ipratropium bromide should to be given with salbutamol for maximum benefit (when indicated). Alternating ipratropium with salbutamol has lesser efficacy than giving them together.
- Steroids rapidly reverse the tachyphylaxis induced by β_2-receptor desensitization which occurs after prolonged β_2-agonist use. Steroids facilitate β_2-agonist bronchodilation action followed by later anti-inflammatory role; hence steroids should be administered early.
- Start steroids if response to bronchodilator is poor. Give to high-risk cases—if patient is steroid dependent, has had recent emergency room visit, previous admission to ICU, severe asthma on high-dose inhaled steroids.
- Titrate terbutaline infusion to desired effect. Monitor ECG, electrolytes, urine analysis and cardiac enzymes.
- The decision to intubate and ventilate a child is usually based on clinical criteria. Respiratory muscle fatigue, exhaustion, diminution of chest expansion, decreased air entry, deterioration of mental status and diaphoresis in recumbent position are clinical indicators of intubation.
- Magnesium is thought to act as a competitive antagonist to calcium mediated smooth muscle constriction. It can be used in severe exacerbations that are refractory to other modalities. Use magnesium sulphate, 25-75 mg/kg/dose IV infused over 20 minutes, every 4-6 hours. Do not use in hypotension or renal failure. Toxicity includes muscle weakness, areflexia and respiratory depression.
- Dehydration is common due to insensible fluid losses and reduced fluid intake. Fluid management is essential in all cases.

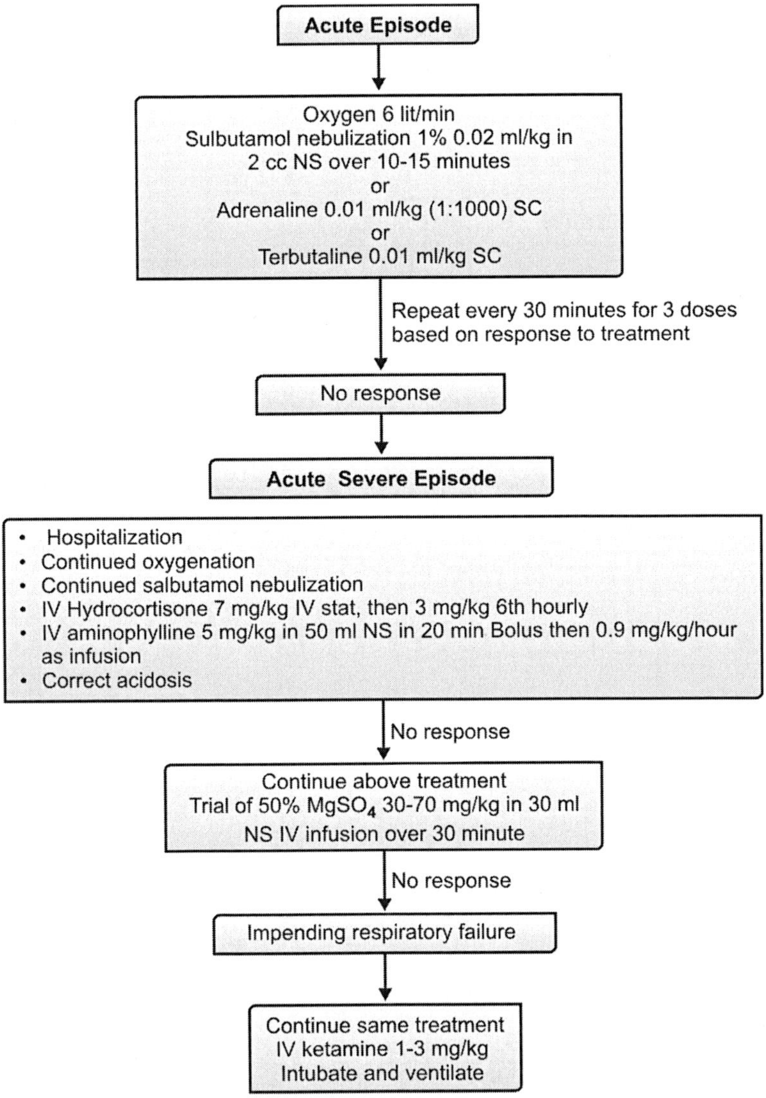

Note:

- Concomitant use of inhaled cholinergics with β_2-agonists causes rapid improvement.
- ABG values alone do not indicate need for mechanical, ventilation and should be interpreted in context of clinical picture.

17

Spontaneous Pneumothorax

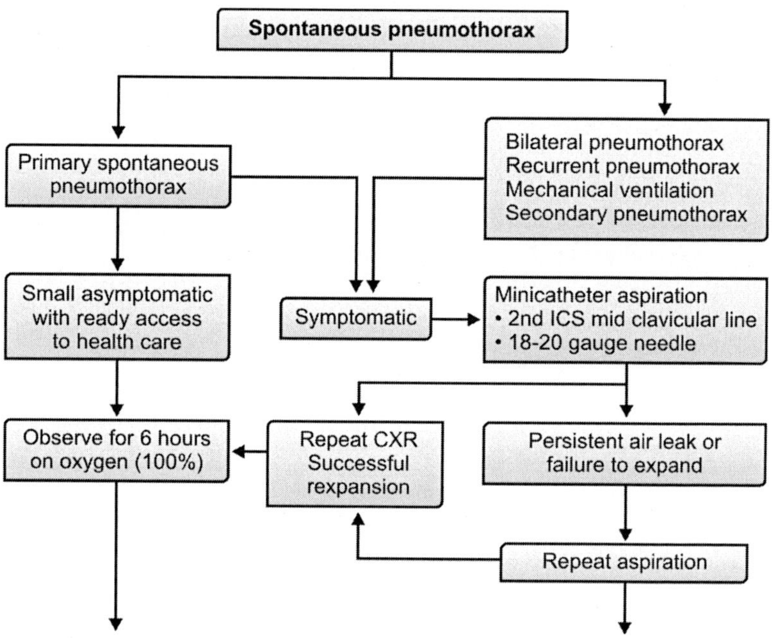

Contd...

Contd...

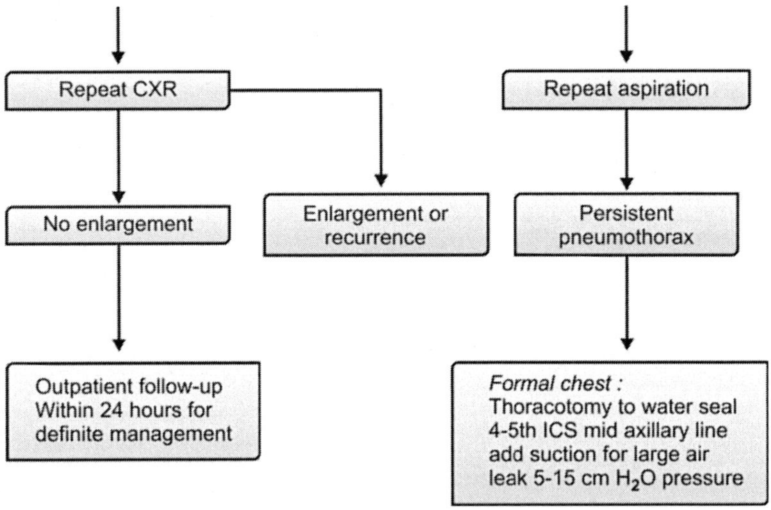
Repeat CXR
No enlargement
Enlargement or recurrence
Outpatient follow-up Within 24 hours for definite management
Repeat aspiration
Persistent pneumothorax
Formal chest :
Thoracotomy to water seal
4-5th ICS mid axillary line
add suction for large air
leak 5-15 cm H_2O pressure

18

Fulminant Hepatic Failure

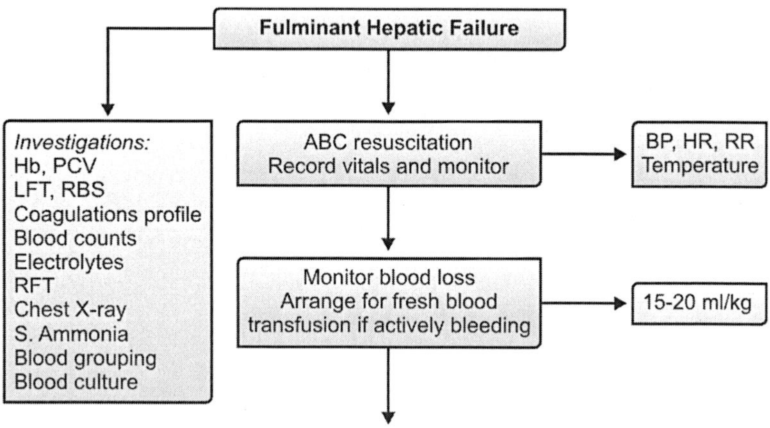

Contd...

Contd...

Drugs

- Inj. Vit K 0.2 mg/kg IV maximum 10 mg/day for 3 days
- Inj. Tanitidine 4-6 mg /kg/day IV 8th hrly
- Bowel wash with lactulose/glucose solutions
- Oral lactulose 0.5 – 1ml/kg 8th hrly
- Oral Neomycin 50-100mg/Kg daily
- Intranenous broad spectrum antibiotics

Fluid Therapy

- 70% of requirement in 1st 24 hours
- Maintenance with daily output + Insensible loss
- Fluid based on Electrolyte status
- 25% Dextrose IV 2 mg/kg/min (maintain blood sugar 100—150 mg%)

Diet

- Restrict protein intake: 0.5 – 1 gm/kg/ day
- Supplement water soluble vitamins

Management of Complications

- Cerebral edema 10% mannitol 5 ml/kg IV bolus–followed by 2 ml/kg 6th hourly
- Coagulopathy: inj. VIt K, Fresh frozen plasma 15 ml/kg
- Convulsions: IV inj. Diazepam, IV Inj. Phenytoin

Note:

- If neomycin is not available may use Streptomycin or Ampicillin
- In cases of paracetamol induced hepatic failure N-acetyl cysteine may be used.

19

Upper Gastrointestinal Bleed

- Intraveneous access with a large bore peripheral line is critical, especially in apparently stable patient in whom shock may be delayed.
- Generally crystalloids are preferred for initial fluid resuscitation.
- Dextran may affect platelet function and should be avoided.
- Use of colloids is reserved for patients with ongoing bleed.
- Overexpansion of intravascular volume is potentially dangerous as it increases risk of rebleeding. After correcting shock, further volume replacement should be titrated to match continuing blood loss.
- In patients with initial signs and symptoms suggestive of 20-25% blood loss, oxygen should be given, consider invasive monitoring to facilitate fluid management.
- Iced-saline lavage has many adverse effects and its efficacy is unproven. Saline or tap water at room temperature is preferred for the purpose of diagnosis and clot removal.

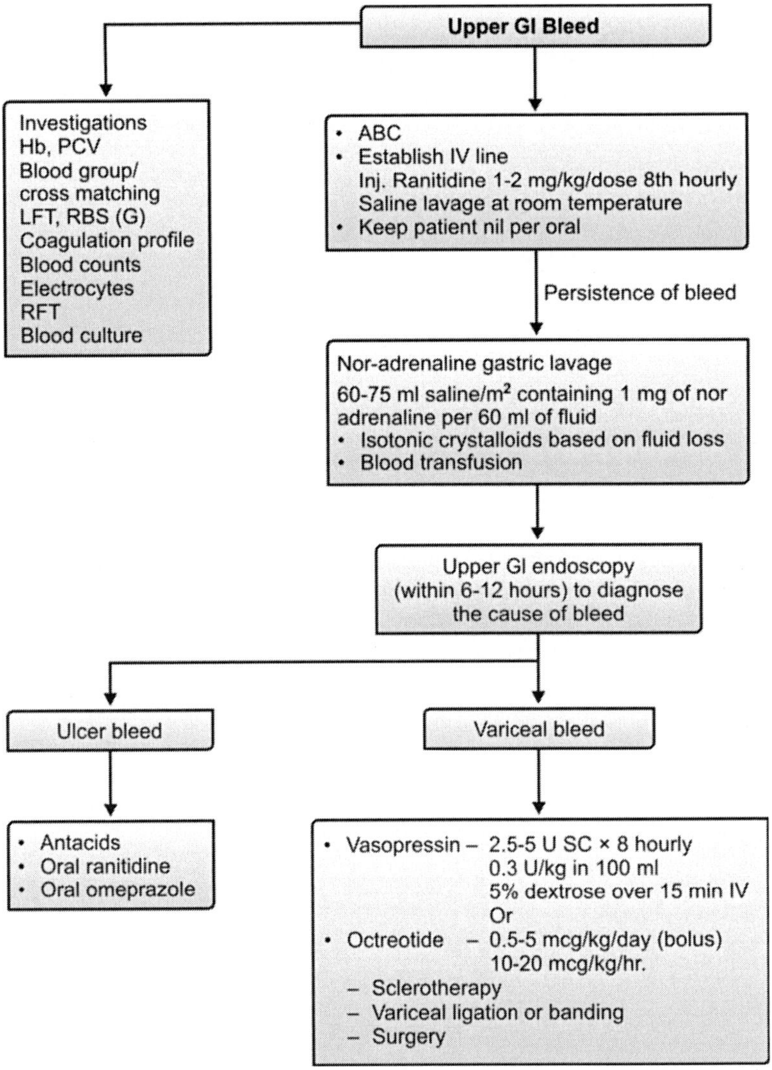
Upper GI Bleed
Investigations
Hb, PCV
Blood group/
cross matching
LFT, RBS (G)
Coagulation profile
Blood counts
Electrocytes
RFT
Blood culture
• ABC
• Establish IV line
Inj. Ranitidine 1-2 mg/kg/dose 8th hourly
Saline lavage at room temperature
• Keep patient nil per oral
Persistence of bleed
Nor-adrenaline gastric lavage
60-75 ml saline/m² containing 1 mg of nor adrenaline per 60 ml of fluid
• Isotonic crystalloids based on fluid loss
• Blood transfusion
Upper GI endoscopy
(within 6-12 hours) to diagnose
the cause of bleed
Ulcer bleed
Variceal bleed
• Antacids
• Oral ranitidine
• Oral omeprazole
• Vasopressin – 2.5-5 U SC × 8 hourly
0.3 U/kg in 100 ml
5% dextrose over 15 min IV
Or
• Octreotide – 0.5-5 mcg/kg/day (bolus)
10-20 mcg/kg/hr.
– Sclerotherapy
– Variceal ligation or banding
– Surgery

20

Acute Renal Failure

Prerenal	*Intrinsic acute renal failure*	*Postrenal acute renal failure*
Hypovolemia	Hypervolemia	UT obstruction
Hypotension	Hypertension	Urine Osmol > 40 mOsm/L
Hypoxia	Drugs/toxins	Urinary Na > 40 mEq/L
Urine Osmol > 500 m Osm/L	Multisystem involvement	Blood urea nitrogen < 20
Blood urea Nitrogen > 20	Urine Osmol < 500 m Osm/L	FeNa > 2
Fe Na < 1	Blood urea nitrogen < 20 FeNa > 2	Specific gravity 1.010
Specific gravity > 1.020	Specific gravity < 1.010	
RFI < 1	RFI >1	

- $\text{FeNa} = \frac{\text{UNa}}{\text{PNa}} \div \frac{\text{UCr}}{\text{PCr}} \times 100$
- $\text{RFI} = \frac{\text{UNa}}{\text{UCr/PCr}}$
- U = Urine, P = Plasma

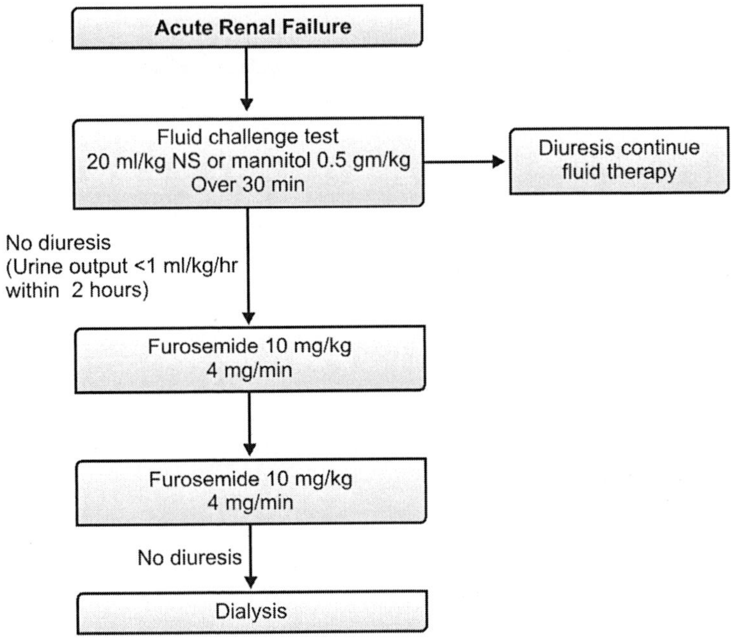

Note:

- Dopamine 2 mcg/kg/min (to improve renal blood flow)
- Correct if present:
  - Electrolyte imbalance—hypocalcemia, hyponatremia
  - Acidosis
  - Hypertension
- Consider etiological management.

21

Management of Hypertension

DRUGS USED IN HYPERTENSION

Vasodilators		
Nifedipine	0.25-2 mg/kg per 24 hrs	2 divided doses
Hydralazine	1-8 mg/kg per 24 hrs	2-3 divided doses
Prazosin	0.05-0.4 mg/kg per 24 hrs	2-3 divided doses
Minoxidil	200 mcg-1.0 mg/kg	Single dose
Beta-blockers		
Propranolol	1-10 mg/kg per 24 hrs	2-3 divided doses
Atenolol	1-4 mg/kg per 24 hrs	Once/day if adequate renal function
Diuretics		
Frusemide	1-5 mg/kg per 24 hrs	1-2 divided doses
Spironolactone	1-3 mg/kg per 24 hrs	1-2 divided doses
ACE inhibitors		
Captopril	0.5-5 mg/kg per 24 hrs	2-3 divided doses
Enalapril	0.1 mg-1 mg/kg per 24 hrs	Single dose

Note:

- The rate of reduction of BP:
  40% in first six hrs
  30% next 12-36 hrs
  30% next 48-96 hrs
- Avoid combination of diuretics and nifedipine.
  Avoid ACE inhibitors in renal artery stenosis.

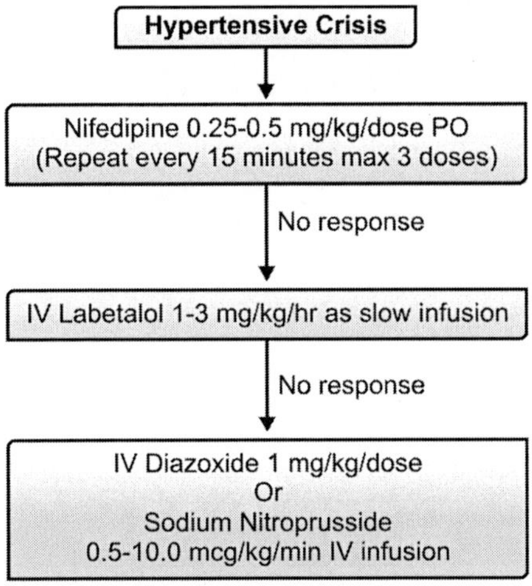

DRUGS USED IN HYPERTENSIVE CRISIS

Drug	*Administration*	*Onset Effect*	*Side Effects*
Nifedipine	Sublingual hourly prn 0.2-0.5 mg/kg	Minutes	Headaches, tachycardia
Sodium Nitroprusside	0.5-10 mcg/kg/ min As infusion	Seconds/minutes	Very rapid effect, titrate dose, cyanide Accumulates after 48 hours of use
Labetalol	1-3 mg/kg/hr	10-30 minutes	Postural hypotension
Hydralazine	Slow IV 0.1-0.5 mg/kg	10-30 minutes	Tachycardia, flushing, headaches
Phentolamine	0.02-0.1 mg/kg	Minutes	Use in catecholamine excess states

22

Status Epilepticus

- Maintaining adequate oxygenation and perfusion is the first priority. Give careful attention to adequency of airway, breathing and circulation.
- Ensure airway patency give 100% O_2.
- Give bag and mask ventilation if there are signs of inadequate oxygenation.
- Establish vascular access, If IV access is not available use intra-osseous, IM or rectal route for drug delivery. Diazepam and lorazepam can be given PR and midazolam can be given IM.
- Evaluation is done simultaneously to find out underlying cause. Take targeted history, rapid physical examination and relevant investigations.
- All benzodiazepines are equally effective in controling seizures.
- Diazepam—Single dose (maximum)
  - 5 mg if < 5 years
  - 10 mg if > 5 years
- Treat the treatable: Lower raised temperature
  - Correct abnormal lab parameters
  - Treat infection if suspected
- In case of raised intracranial tension
  - Treat with inj. Mannitol

- 2/3rd of maintenance fluid
- consider CT scan after stabilization

- Be ready to intubate at any stage of management.

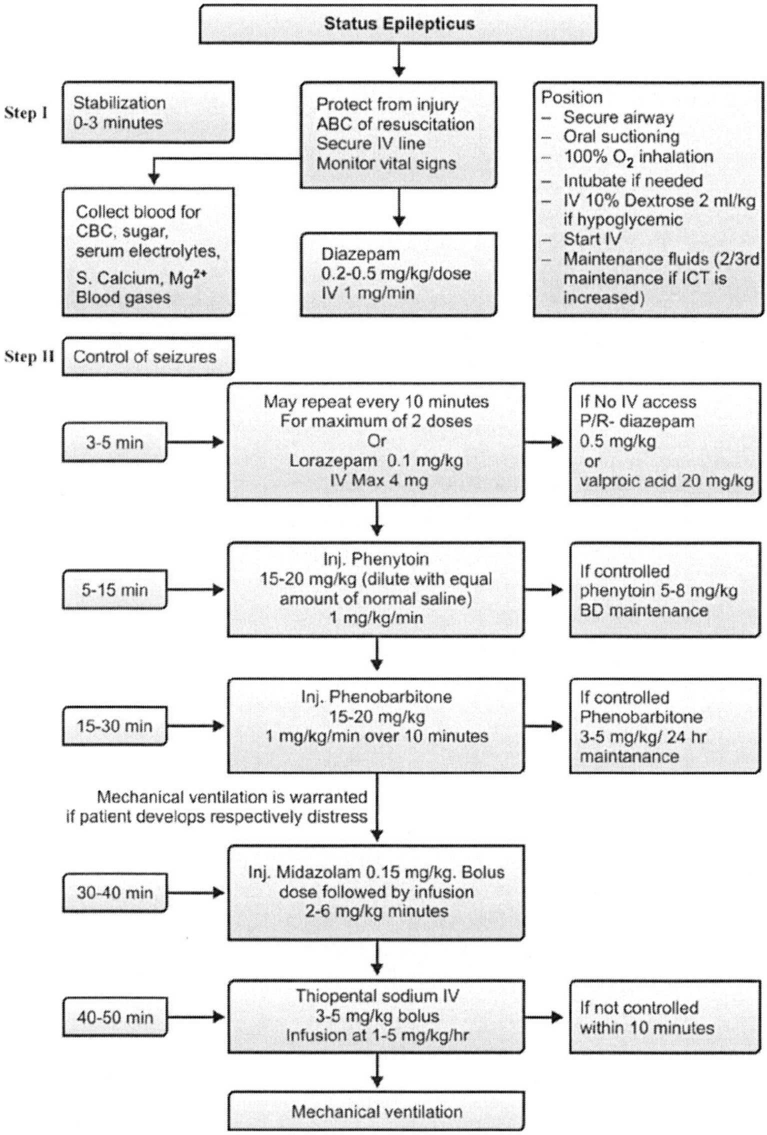

23

Coma

Note the following causes while evaluation

- Consider other infections
  Bacterial, viral, rickettsial, parasites
- Vascular—Vasculitis
  - Hypertensive encephalopathy
- Epilepsy—Postictal
  - Non-convulsive status epilepticus
- Toxic—Endogenous – liver/renal
  - Exogenous – Insect bite
  - Substance abuses
  - Drugs/Poisons
- Metabolic—Glucose, electrolytes and acid base disturbance
  - Hyperammonemia
  - Inborn errors of metabolism
  - Reye's syndrome
- Endocrine—Hypothyroidism, adrenal failure
- Hypoxic—Ischemia
- Hysterical coma
  - Adolescent children (girls)
  - Voluantary closure of eyelid during passive opening of eyelids
  - Nystagmus after calorie stimulation

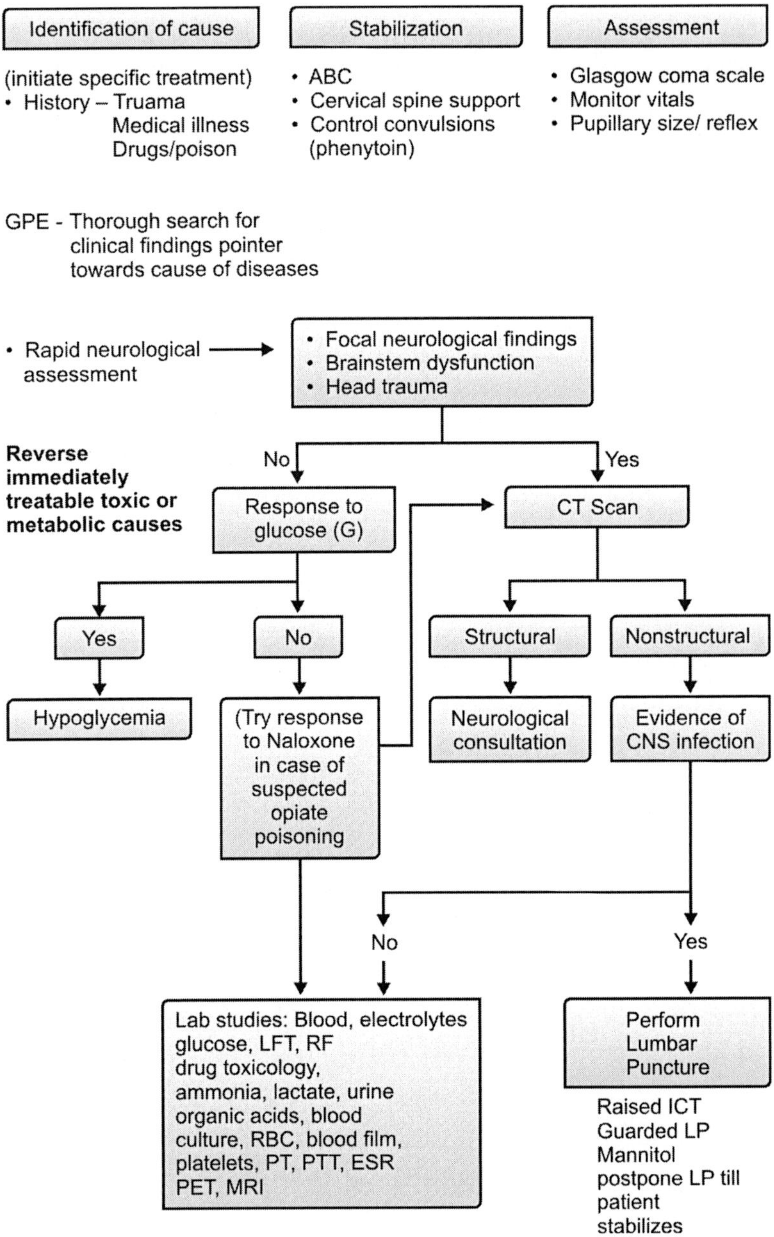
Identification of cause
(initiate specific treatment)
• History – Truama
Medical illness
Drugs/poison
Stabilization
• ABC
• Cervical spine support
• Control convulsions (phenytoin)
Assessment
• Glasgow coma scale
• Monitor vitals
• Pupillary size/ reflex
GPE - Thorough search for clinical findings pointer towards cause of diseases
• Rapid neurological assessment
• Focal neurological findings
• Brainstem dysfunction
• Head trauma
Reverse immediately treatable toxic or metabolic causes
No
Yes
Response to glucose (G)
CT Scan
Yes
No
Structural
Nonstructural
Hypoglycemia
(Try response to Naloxone in case of suspected opiate poisoning
Neurological consultation
Evidence of CNS infection
No
Yes
Lab studies: Blood, electrolytes glucose, LFT, RF drug toxicology, ammonia, lactate, urine organic acids, blood culture, RBC, blood film, platelets, PT, PTT, ESR PET, MRI
Perform Lumbar Puncture
Raised ICT
Guarded LP
Mannitol
postpone LP till patient stabilizes

24

Disseminated Intravascular Coagulation

Disseminated Intravascular Coagulation (DIC)

Lab investigations:
Hb
Peripheral smear
BT, CT
PT, APTT
Platelet count
Fibrin spilt products
Fibrinogen levels
Serum electrolytes

- Oxygen
- Monitor vital parameters
- IV fluids
- Correct shock – 20 ml/kg NS/ RL
- Dopamine
- Correct electrolyte imbalance and acidosis
- Inj. vitamin K.

Correct anemia ⟶ Packed RBC (15 ml/kg body weight)
Thrombocytopenia ⟶ Platelet concentrates
Coagulopathy ⟶ Fresh frozen plasma (15 ml/kg)
Cryoprecipitate (1 unit/10 kg)
Heparin therapy ⟶ 15 units/kg/hour as continuous infusion
Start specific treatment for correction of underlying condition

25

Management of Blood Transfusion Reactions

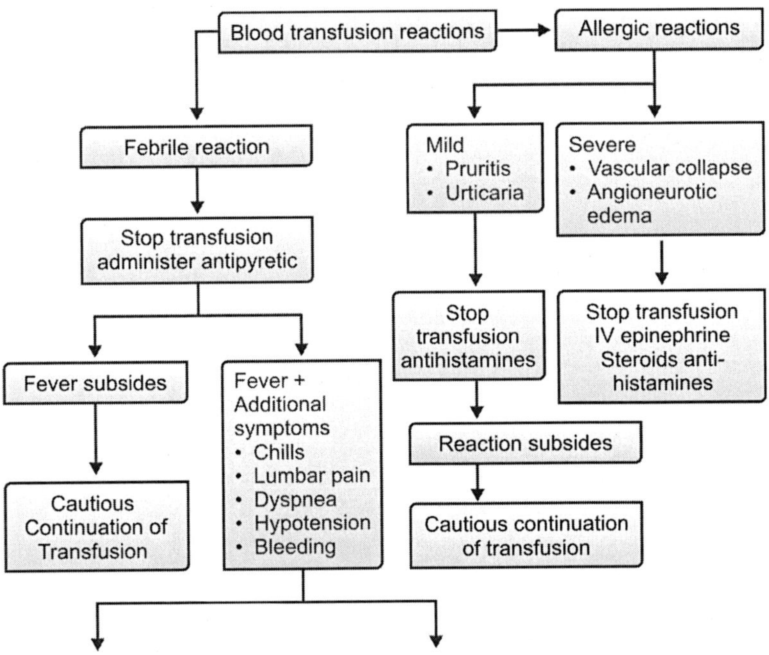

Contd...

Contd...

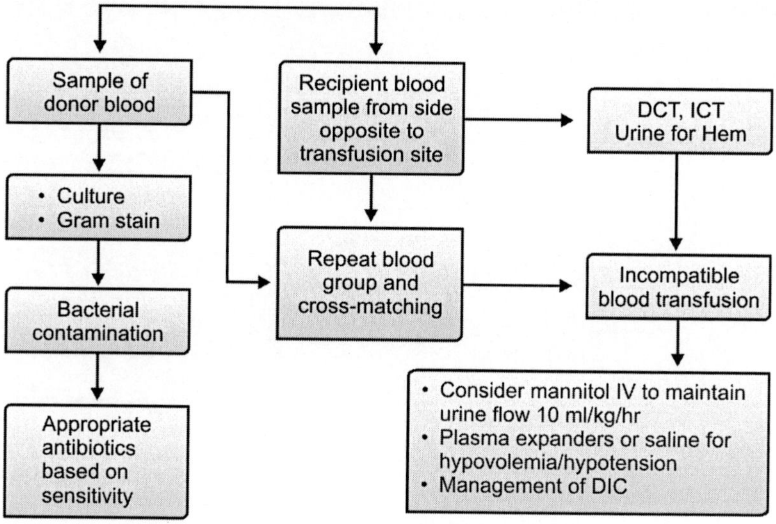

Note: *Adrenaline*: 0.01 ml/kg/ dose of 1:1000 solution SC
Repeat dose after 15-20 minutes

Mannitol: 5 ml/kg of 20% solution IV bolus. 2 ml /kg 6th hourly IV thereafter.

Antihistamine: Pheniramine maleate: 0.5 mg/kg/day Q 8th hourly IM or IV.

26

Hyponatremia

- Hyponatremia is not a disease but a manifestation of variety of disorders.
- Most cases of hyponatremia are associated with a low plasma osmolality, either due to primary Na^+ loss or primary water gain.
- Clinical features of hyponatremia are related to osmotic water shift leading to increased ICF volume,especially cerebral edema.
- Severity of clinical features depends on the rapidity of onset and absolute decrease in plasma sodium concentration.
- Adaptive mechanisms designed to protect cell volume occur in chronic hyponatremia.
- Laboratory findings often give useful information in differential diagnosis—plasma and urine osmolality, urine Na^+ and K^+ concentration.
- Goals of therapy are to raise Na^+ by restricting water intake and promoting water loss and to correct underlying disorder.
- Rate of correction depends on the absence or presence of neurological symptoms.
- In asymptomatic hyponatremia rate of correction should not be more than 10-12 mmol/L over first 24 hours.
- Acute or severe hyponatremia ($Na^+ < 110$-115) requires more rapid correction.

- Severe hyponatremia should be treated with hypertonic saline and plasma Na^+ increased by 1-2 mmol/hour for first 3-4 hours till seizures subside. After this rate of correction should be 0.5-1 mmol/hour.

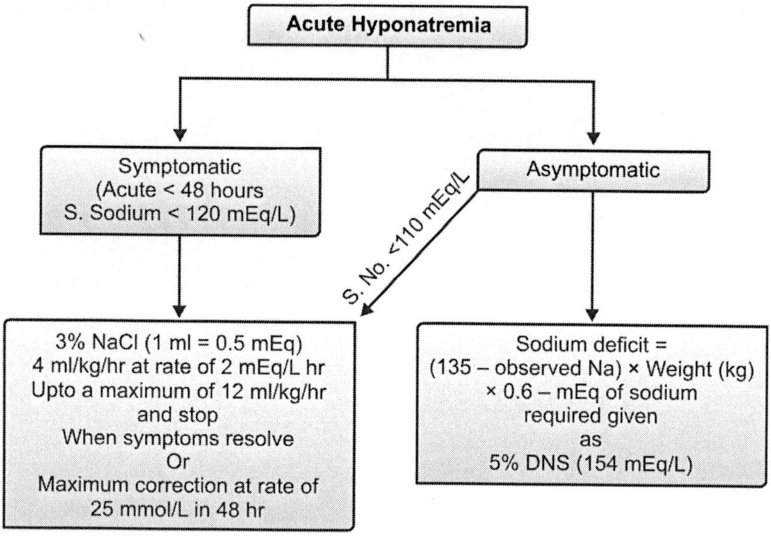

27

Hypernatremia

- Majority of cases result from loss of water.
- Source of free water loss is either renal or extrarenal (Evaporation from skin, respiratory tract, GI loss)
- Clinical features are related to hypertonicity which leads to contracted ICF volume and decreased brain-cell volume.
- Measurement of urinary volume and osmolality are essential in evaluation. Appropriate renal response indicates extrarenal causes.
- Calculate water deficit
- Water deficit = $\frac{\text{plasma Na}^{+}\text{ conc} - 140 * \text{TBW}}{140}$

  where, TBW = Total body water
- Rapid correction is dangerous as it leads to cellular edema.
- Ongoing water losses should be taken into account while replacing water.
- Safest route of administration of water is by mouth or via NG tube.

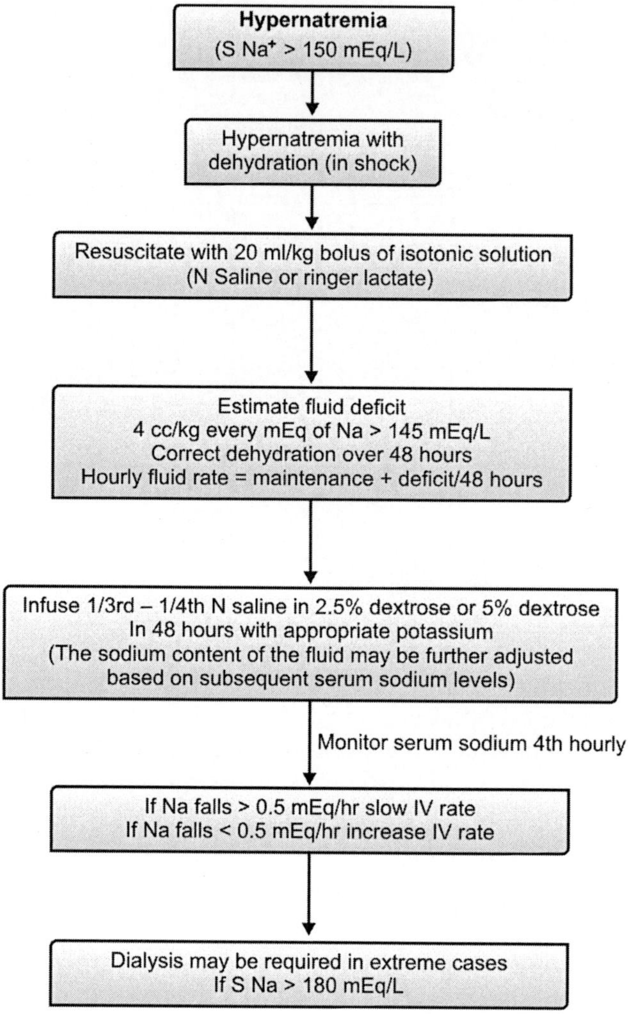

Note:

- Hypernatremia correction should reduce sodium at 0.5 mEq/L/hr (12 mEq/L/day).
- Do not correct water deficit rapidly with sodium solutions (NS) as it causes severe sodium overload and cerebral edema.
- Treatment depending on the cause.

28

Hypokalemia

- A low K^+ concentration may result from decreased K^+ intake, increased K^+ losses (Renal or GI), shift of K^+ from extracellular fluid to intracellular fluid.
- The relationship between serum K^+ concentration and total body K^+ content has no definite correlation and there is no readily available method of determining total body K^+ loss.
- Hypokalemia leads to impaired neuronal impulse transmission and muscular contractions.
- Potassium chloride is preferable salt since it replinishes chloride and corrects the alkalosis associated with hypokalemia.
- If serum K^+ concentration is < 2.5 mmol/L, a dose of 0.5 mEq/kg of potassium chloride is infused over 30 minutes with continuous ECG monitoring may be safely used in children except in the settings of shock, oliguria or acidosis.
- Potassium chloride should not be pushed intravenously due to risk of ventricular fibrillation.
- Patients with DKA should get potassium phosphate to prevent the hypokalemia and phosphate depletion.

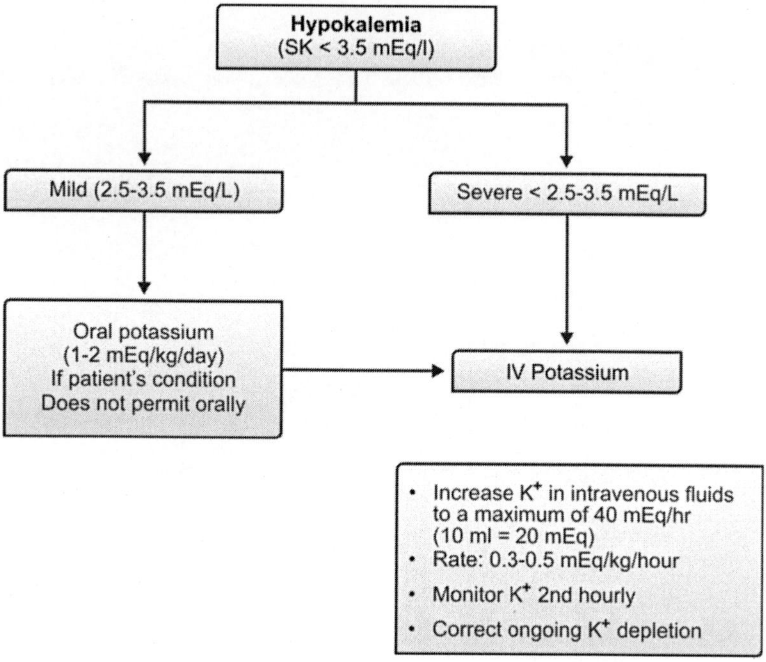

Note: Higher concentration of > 40 mEq/L of potassium if required should be tried only through central line because potassium solutions are highly irritant to peripheral vein.

29

Hyperkalemia

- *β_2 agonist* – Salbutamol – 0.05 ml/kg/nebulization
  Onset of action: 10-20 min
  Mechanism: Intracellular K^+ shift
- *Sodium bicarbonate*—1-2 mEq/kg over 10 min
  Onset: 20 minutes
  Duration of action 1-4 hours
  Mode of action: Results in intracellular K^+ shift
- *Calcium gluconate* (10%)—0.5 ml/kg/over 10 minutes may be repeated twice
  Onset: Immediate
  Duration: 30-60 minutes
  Mode of action: Myocardial protection (Physiological antagonist)
- *Glucose-insulin*: 1 gm/kg dextrose + 0.1 unit/kg insulin as infusion over 1 hour
  Or 25% dextrose 50 ml + 2-3 units insulin
  Give 1-2 ml/kg over 10-20 minutes, then at 4-8 ml/kg/hr
  Onset: 15-30 minutes
  Mode of action: Insulin causes intracellular shift of potassium
- *Kayexalate (Sodium resonium Or Calcium resonium)*—
  1 gm/kg PR or via nasogastric tube
  Onset: 30-60 minutes
  Mode of action: Decreases body K^+ by exchanging Na^+ for K^+ (Sodium resonium)

- *Frusemide (in nonanureic patients)—*
  1-2 mg/kg IV
  Mechanism: Increased urinary excretion of K^+
  Dialysis: Hemodialysis more efficient
  (hemodialysis or rapid cycling, peritoneal dialysis)
  Mechanism: Removes K^+ from body

Note:

- Avoid all potassium rich food.
  For example, fruits, tender coconut water
- Avoid nephrotoxic drugs. Modify drug dosage and frequency depending on renal parameters.

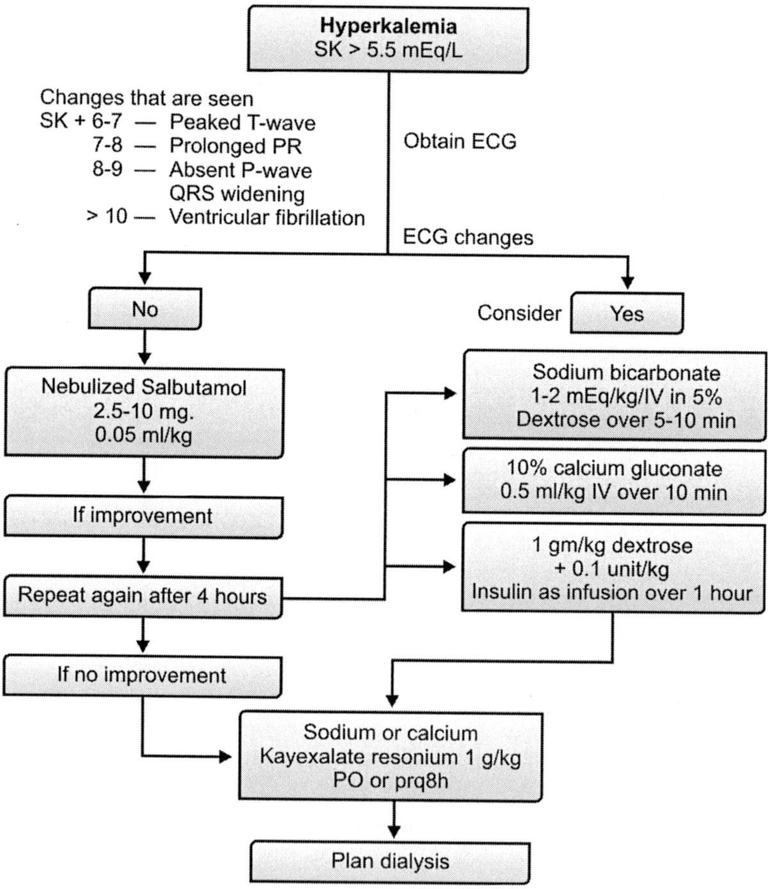

30

Diabetic Ketoacidosis

- Slowly correcting fluid deficit over 24-48 hrs appears safer than rapid rehydration.
- In a child with severe acidosis or compromised circulation, initial volume resuscitation can be administered over 30 minutes. After that slowly correct water deficit by providing normal maintenance fluids plus calculated deficits.
- After initial fluid bolus the rate of infusion (ml/hour) for next 23 hours = [Calculated fluid for 24 hrs – Ist hour bolus]/23.
- Greater risk of cerebral edema is seen in patients who received insulin in the first hour. Insulin is usually started after fluid resuscitation.
- Glucose levels should not fall faster than 50-100 mg per hour. Infusion rate can be reduced as glucose levels fall but should be maintained above 0.05 U/kg/hr (minimum rate required to prevent ketosis)
- Do not discontinue infusion until subcutaneous insulin is given
- After initial resuscitation if serum sodium level is low, "pseudohyponatremia" is often present. Corrected Na = measured Na^+ 1.6 [(glucose – 100)/100]. If the value exceeds 150 mEq/L, duration of fluid correction should be extended to 36 hours and bolus volume replacement if needed in between

should be with 1/2 NS. During treatment sodium level rises. If sodium does not rise, true hyponatremia may be present. This may increase cerebral edema risk and should be treated.

- Hypokalemia should be anticipated, detected and corrected at the earliest. Easy assessment is by a cardiac monitor or by ECG in Lead II. Earliest evidence is flat T waves (< 2 div) followed by the appearance U wave and QRS widening. To correct hypokalemia add potassium chloride to IV fluid up to 40 mEq/L even, if the child has not passed urine. Insulin infusion should be postponed till the correction of hypokalemia in such patients. Infusion rates of potassium;
  - Sr. potassium < 2.5, give 1 mEq/kg body weight by separate infusion over 1 hour.

    2.5-3.5 add 40 mEq/L
    3.5-5 add 20 mEq/L
    5-6 add 10 mEq/L (optional).
    > 6 mEq, stop potassium and repeat test in two hours.
- If there is no evidence of hypokalemia potassium should be withheld till the child has voided. Calcium (50 mg/kg/day) and phosphorus (25 mg/kg/day) should be started as soon as child tolerates oral.
- Excessive use of fluids, use of bicarbonate and large doses of insulin have been linked to formation of cerebral edema.
- Avoid bicarbonate to treat acidosis. Ketoacidosis gets corrected with fluid and insulin infusion. Failure of acidosis to improve with treatment reflects inadequate fluid and insulin replacement. The definite indications for bicarbonate therapy are symptomatic hyperkalemia, (revealed by tented T waves in ECG and cardiac irregularity), circulatory failure and renal failure. Blood pH < 7 without clinical signs of organ function impairment is not a definite indication. Dose of bicarbonate is 0.5-1 mEq/kg (max 50 mEq) in 1:1 dilution in sterile water to be administered in 60 minutes through separate IV line. Rebound hypokalemia and cerebral edema should be anticipated.
- Till recovery maintain a flowchart for proper follow-up. Vitals, GCS, Pupil size, BG, ECG, insulin dose and I/O chart are to be monitored hourly till BG is 250 mg/dL. Thereafter all

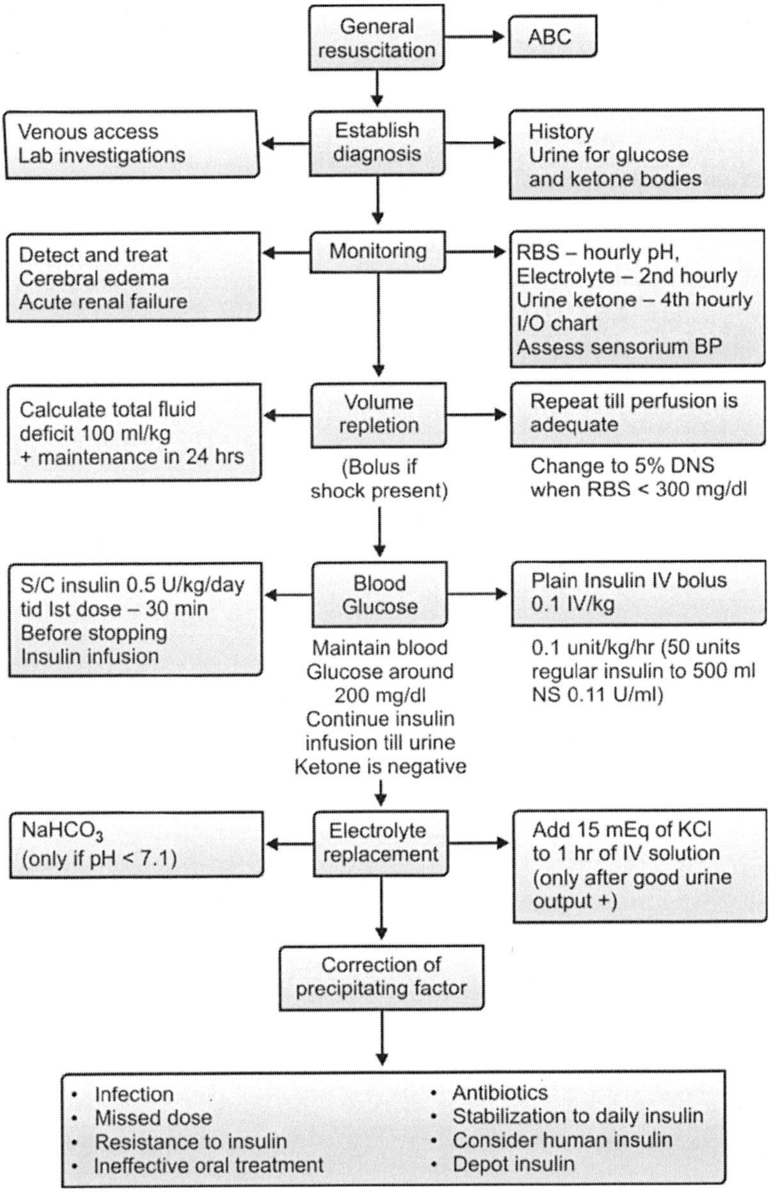
General resuscitation
ABC
Establish diagnosis
Venous access
Lab investigations
History
Urine for glucose
and ketone bodies
Monitoring
Detect and treat
Cerebral edema
Acute renal failure
RBS – hourly pH,
Electrolyte – 2nd hourly
Urine ketone – 4th hourly
I/O chart
Assess sensorium BP
Volume repletion
(Bolus if shock present)
Calculate total fluid
deficit 100 ml/kg
+ maintenance in 24 hrs
Repeat till perfusion is adequate
Change to 5% DNS
when RBS < 300 mg/dl
Blood Glucose
Maintain blood
Glucose around
200 mg/dl
Continue insulin
infusion till urine
Ketone is negative
S/C insulin 0.5 U/kg/day
tid Ist dose – 30 min
Before stopping
Insulin infusion
Plain Insulin IV bolus
0.1 IV/kg
0.1 unit/kg/hr (50 units
regular insulin to 500 ml
NS 0.11 U/ml)
Electrolyte replacement
NaHCO3
(only if pH < 7.1)
Add 15 mEq of KCl
to 1 hr of IV solution
(only after good urine
output +)
Correction of precipitating factor
• Infection
• Missed dose
• Resistance to insulin
• Ineffective oral treatment
• Antibiotics
• Stabilization to daily insulin
• Consider human insulin
• Depot insulin

parameters except BG need be monitored 4-6 hourly. BG should be monitored hourly till the child is stable and free of acidosis. Blood gas (pH, PCO_2, HCO_3) and electrolytes (Na, K, Cl, and HCO_3) need be evaluated 4 hourly. Urine glucose and acetone are to be evaluated 4 hourly or with each void. Mannitol should be kept ready to counter act cerebral edema. Spuriously high level of serum creatinine can occur without renal failure in ketoacidosis.

- Indications for discontinuing IV fluids are correction of dehydration, child stable on oral feeds, venous pH > 7.3, S Na 135-145 mEq/L and clearance of ketonuria.
- Other management includes coma care, detection and treatment of infections (especially vulvovaginitis), frequent monitoring, re-evaluation of clinical and lab parameters and individualized alteration in protocol. Less severe cases will be fit for early weaning from IV fluids and continuous IV insulin infusion may not be required.

31

Poisoning: General Guidelines

- Decontaminate—remove clothing, wash with soap and water. Rinse the eye for 10-15 minutes.
- Ensure ABC
- Emesis*/gastric lavage < 4 h.
  Most effective < 1 hour of ingestion.
  Syp. Ipecac > 6 months-12 years, 10-15 ml followed by water
  If no emesis by 30 minutes
  Repeat 2nd dose
  Maximum 2 doses

- *Cathartics*
  - Cathartics—sorbitol (70%) 1 ml/kg
  - Avoid: Magnesium cathartics in renal disease.
  - Sodium cathartics in CCF and hypertension.

- Prevent GI absorption
  - Activated charcoal
    Children < 1 year 1 gm/kg
    Children < 1-12 years 25-50 gm.

> *** Note:**
> - Late emesis/gastric lavage is
> - Useful in anticholinergics,
> - Narcotics, salicylates.
> - *Emesis/gastric lavage is contraindicated*
> - Patient is convulsing
>   - Comatosed
>   - Hematemesis
> - Kerosene ingestion
> - Corrosive ingestion

  - Adolescents 25-100 gm.
- Avoid in acids, alkalis, cyanides, iron ingestion
  - Mix charcoal in 8-10 times the amount of water.
  - If possible give the whole amount at once. If the child has difficulty in tolerating it, the dose can be divided.
- Albumin water or milk
- Total bowel irrigation
  Avoid in lleus, bowel performation, GI obstruction
- *Eliminate poison*
  Forced alkaline diuresis useful in salicylates and barbiturates poisoning
- Use specific antidotes.

Abnormal Color of Urine

Gives clue to the type of poison ingested.
- Blue or green—Methylene blue.
- Orange—Rifampicin, iron poisoning treated with desferroxamine.
- Grey or black—Phenols or cresols.
- *$FeCl_3$ test*: Positive for salicylate poisoning, phenothiazines, PAS, INH.

Note:
- Check the child for emergency signs at admission and treat accordingly. Check for hypoglycemia.
- Identify the specific agent and remove or adsorb it as soon as possible.
- Never use salt as an emetic as this can be fatal.
- Perform gastric lavage with 10 ml/kg body weight of warm normal saline.
- Keep the child under observation for 4-24 hours depending on the poison swallowed.
- Give supplemental O_2 if required and also in inhaled poisons.

32

Organophosphorus Poisoning

Organophosphorus Poisoning

↓

Remove from site of exposure remove clothing

↓

Wash skin with soap and water

↓

Administration of activated charcoal

↓

In severely affected patients ventilation

↓

Atropine

- 0.05 mg/kg IM or by IV infusion over 15 minutes, every 10-15 min
- Until oral and bronchial secretions becomes dry
- Decrease frequency to Q 30-60 minutely and further max 12 mg/24 hours (Atropine infusion 0.02 mg/kg/hr also effective)

Pralidoxime (PAM)

- 20-40 mg/kg over 30 min in normal saline over 30 minutes
- Repeat after one hour if symptoms persist
- Repeat Q 6-8 hourly 24-48 hrs until all nicotinic symptoms ablated

Note:

- Pralidoxime to be given preferably within 12 hours (contraindicated in carbamate poisoning).
- Pupillary response is not an indication of atropinization.
- Tachycardia not a contraindication for atropine.
- Give activated charcoal if organophosphorus compound is ingested and within 1 hr of the ingestion.
- Do not induce vomiting because most pesticides are in petrol based solvents.
- Careful aspiration of stomach contents by NG tube can be done in serious ingestion where activated charcoal cannot be given (The airway should be protected).
- Check for hypoxia with pulse oxymetry. Atropine can cause ventricular arrhythmias in hypoxic children.
- Give pralidoxime if there is muscle weakness. Give bolus followed by an IV infusion of 10-20 mg/kg/hr or repeated doses every 6-8 hours as necessary.

33

Hydrocarbon Poisoning

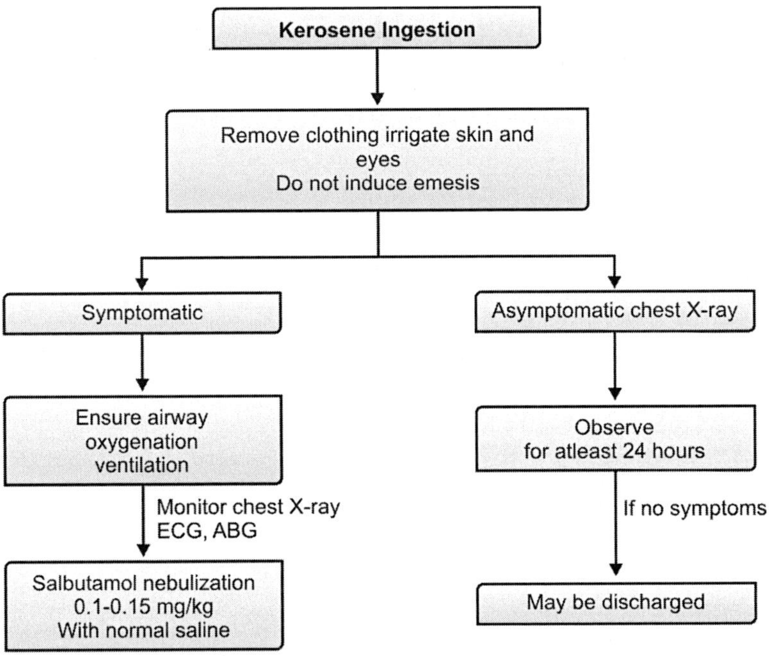

SUPPORTIVE MANAGEMENT IS THE MAINSTAY OF TREATMENT

- Antibiotics are recommended only if associated with lower respiratory tract infection.
- Gastric lavage may be useful for large recent ingestion but the airway may need protection with a cuffed endotracheal tube.
- Beneficial role of activated charcoal is not clear cut.

34

Scorpion Envenomation

Local Care →	Tourniquet application Proximal to the sting to delay absorption of toxins
→	2% lignocaine for pain relief
Systemic Care →	Prazocin—0.4 mg/kg in 2-3 divided doses
→	Ranitidine 1-2 mg/kg/dose IV 2-4 mg/kg/day oral
→	Insulin 0.1 units/kg/dose subcutaneously Q 8 h for myocardial protection
→	Captopril 0.5-1.0 mg/kg/dose If hypertension persists despite prazocin

Note:

- Steroids, lytic cocktail, digoxin have no role and are contraindicated.
- If the patient develops pulmonary edema, supportive care with IV furosemide, assisted ventilation.
- Give paracetamol or other drugs for adequate pain relief. If pain is very severe, infiltrate sting site with 1% lignocaine, without epinephrine.

35

Snakebite

FIRST AID

- Tourniquet
  - For bites on extremities within 1 hour of bite
  - Apply band 1 inch wide, 5 cm above fang marks or upper limit of edema
  - Should admit one finger between band and skin thus ensuring only obstruction of lymphatic drainage and not venous return.
- Reassurance
- Immobilize the limb
- Clean the would, avoid cutting the wound.
- Polyvalent antisnake venom after test for sensitivity
  (In case of signs of envenomation start ASV without test dose under cover of steroids and antihistamines keeping preloaded adrenaline ready)
- *In case of CNS symptoms:*
  Inj. Neostigmine 0.07 mg/kg IV Q 6 hrly.
  Inj. Atropine 20-50 mcg/kg
- In case of respiratory paralysis: Mechanical ventilation
- Correct shock if present—Isotonic saline 20 ml/kg
- Investigations: Monitor BT, CT, Hb, Coagulation profile, Platelet count, LFT, RFT, TC, DC, blood group, cross-matching, urine analysis, ECG.

- If actively bleeding—transfuse fresh blood 15-20 ml/kg.
- *Wound management*:
  - Clean the wound with sterile saline
  - Inj. tetanus toxoid (if not immunized/received toxoid within the last five years).
  - Pain relief, start broad spectrum antibiotics, fluid management.

Severity of envenomation	*Clinical features*	*Approx. dose of ASV*
Mild	Progressive local swelling, local purpura Ecchymosis	5 vials
Moderate	Swelling beyond bite site, Nausea, vomiting and bradycardia hematological changes	5-15 vials
Severe	Extensive local effect Hemolysis, DIC, distant purpura and petechae Shock, encephalopathy, paralysis	15-20 vials

Note:
- Test dose of AV- 0.02 ml of 1:100- solution subcutaneously. A positive reaction may manifest within 30 minutes as a wheal.
- ASV is given as continuous infusion diluted in normal saline. (2 vials in 100 ml isotonic saline for mild, 4 vials in 100 ml isotonic saline for moderate/severe evenomation in one hour)
  - Same dose to be repeated over 4 hours until neurological and hematological assessment normalizes.
  - Once neurological and hematological assessment normalizes, last 2 vials of ASV to be administered intravenously over 24 hours in 500 ml normal saline.
- In case of sensitivity to ASV, ASV to be given with Inj. Adrenaline 0.01 ml/kg 1 : 1000 solution subcutaneous to be repeated 15-20 minutes, Inj. pheniramine maleate 0.5 mg/kg/day Q 8th hourly IM or IV.
- Seek surgical help for excision of dead tissue to relieve compartment syndrome, for skin grafting and for tracheostomy.

36

Arterial Blood Gas Analysis in Clinical Practice

Knowledge of arterial blood gas (ABG) analysis is important for every clinician who is treating critically ill-patients. ABG analysis reveals oxygenation status, adequacy of ventilation and acid-base balance. It plays a significant role in documenting and monitoring respiratory failure, especially during ventilator and oxygen therapy.

NORMAL METABOLISM AND ITS DYSFUNCTION

Cellular function is ultimately dependent on regular supply of glucose, oxygen and water—consequently, volatile acid like carbonic acid and fixed acids like sulphuric acid, lactic acid and keto acid are constantly poured into the general circulation. Respiratory system plays an important role in eliminating volatile acids while renal mechanisms eliminate fixed acids in the form of hydrogen ions. In pathological states, this homeostasis gets disturbed causing accumulation of the above acids; and resulting in acid-base disturbance. Though renal and respiratory systems take the brunt to overcome acid-base disturbance, the other important mechanism for immediate rescue is the buffer-base system.

Acid/Alkali Balance Equation

In the blood, bicarbonate reacts with hydrogen ions to produce CO_2 and H_2O

$$H^+ + HCO_3^- \rightleftarrows H_2O + CO_2$$

Normal hydrogen ion concentration in our body is 40 mEq/L (range is 36-44 mEq/L)

Harmful effects of excessive accumulation of hydrogen ions is overcome by body buffer and the respiratory systems (within hours). Renal compensation plays a major role, though it is a delayed process. Water plays an important role by transporting hydrogen ions in nontoxic form. Carbonic anhydrate converts excess of hydrogen ions to CO_2 and eliminates the same through the lungs. Similarly, the excessive accumulation of CO_2. is removed by kidney as hydrogen ion.

$PaCO_2$ (Normal 4.7-6.0 KPa, 36-44 mm Hg)

This is a good indicator of ventilatory adequacy because it is inversely proportional to alveolar minute volume. When the pH is known it can be used to determine primary or compensatory ventilatory changes. When $PaCO_2$ is above the normal value (> 44 mm Hg) respiratory academia results which is designed as ventilatory failure and a decrease of $PaCO_2$ (< 36 mm Hg) results in respiratory alkalosis. For every 20 mm Hg, increase of $PaCO_2$, pH falls by 0.1 unit and for every 10 mm of Hg fall of $PaCO_2$, pH increases by 0.1.

Hydrogen Ion Concentration and Bicarbonate

At normal H^+ ion concentration of 40 mEq/L (pH 7.4), HCO_3^- levels and the range is 22-26. When the HCO_3 level falls below 22 mEq/L metabolic acidosis results. When the HCO_3 levels exceeds 26 mEq/L it is termed as metabolic alkalosis.

pH (Normal 7.36-7.44)

pH is the negative logarithm of hydrogen ion concentration. Normal pH is 7.4 which is equivalent to concentration of 40 mEq/L and the range is 7.36- 7.44. if the pH is near normal it may be due to respiratory or metabolic compensation. This compensation is never complete, so if the pH is near normal it will still always tell you if the child has a compensated acidosis (pH slightly lower than normal) or a compensated alkalosis (pH slightly higher than normal).

Relation of pH with CO_2 and Bicarbonate

The pH of our body ultimately depends upon the levels of $PaCO_2$ and HCO_3 derived by Henderson-Hasselbach equation.

$$pH = \frac{\text{Renal compensation}}{\text{Pulmonary compensation}}$$

$$pH = \frac{6.1 + \log(HCO_3^-)}{0.03 \times PCO_3}$$

Base Excess / Deficit

A positive base excess indicates a metabolic alkalosis. A negative base excess or base deficit indicates metabolic acidosis. A negative base excess is only treated if it is more negative than – 6 and the pH is low.

PaO_2: (normal 10.6 KPa, > 80 mm Hg in air) The normal partial pressure of O_2 in the arterial blood (PaO_2) is 80-100 mm of Hg. When fraction of the inspired O_2 (FiO_2) concentration increases, the arterial PaO_2 increases by five times ($PaO_2 = FiO_2 \times 5$). When PaO_2 falls below 80 mm of Hg hypoxemia results which can be classified as either mild (PaO_2 of 60-80 mm), moderate (PaO_2 of 40-60 mm) or severe (PaO_2 < 40 mm). The tolerance of hypoxemia is better at extremes of ages. In newborn baby, the normal PaO_2 is 40-70 mm of Hg.

SaO_2: Though estimation of PaO_2 through ABG is the best investigation to identify oxygenation status and acid-base disturbances, it requires arterial puncture every time. There is a constant relationship exists between PaO_2 and oxygen saturation of Hb.

PaO_2 40 mm of Hg = SaO_2 70%
PaO_2 50 mm of Hg = SaO_2 80%
PaO_2 60 mm of Hg = SaO_2 90%

Monitoring of SaO_2 is done using pulse oximetry. But it has its own limitations. As higher oxygen tension, poor perfusion status and in methemoglobinemia, pulse oximetry fails.

STAGES OF COMPENSATION

Primary Disturbance	*pH*	*HCO_3*	*PCO_2*
Metabolic Acidosis			
Acute	↓	↓	N
Partially compensation	↓	↓	↓
Fully compensated	N	↓	↓
Respiratory Acidosis			
Acute	↓	N	↑
Partially compensation	↓	↑	↑
Fully compensated	N	↑	↑
Respiratory Alkalosis			
Acute	↑	N	↓
Partially compensation	↑	↓	↓
Fully compensated	N	↓	↓
Metabolic alkalosis			
Acute	↑	↑	N
Partially compensation	↑	↑	↑
Fully compensated	N	↑	↑

Acid-base Disorders

Disturbance of the relationship of HCO_3 with H_2CO_3 results in four simple acid base disorders namely metabolic acidosis, metabolic alkalosis, respiratory acidosis and respiratory alkalosis. In simple disorders both PCO_2 and HCO_3 change in the same direction.

Among the 4 simple disorders metabolic acidosis is common. In some clinical conditions, these simple disorders may coexist resulting in a mixed disorder, when both PCO_2 and HCO_3 are either reduced or increased resulting in near normal pH, though the clinical situation is actually ominous.

(For example, coexistence of metabolic acidosis with respiratory alkalosis in salicylate poisoning).

Buffers and Physiological Compensation

The ultimate aim of the body is to maintain the pH within near normal limits. Extracellular buffers are the first line defense (act within minutes) and include bicarbonate and serum proteins. Intracellular buffers act at a slower rate (within hours) and include intracellular proteins, phosphates and hemoglobin. When chemical buffering is not enough, physiological compensation starts.

When HCO_3 loss occurs form the body (primary event) the respiratory system comes to rescue by eliminating CO_2 (compensatory) form the body quickly (12-24 hrs) till the pH approach normal value. Similarly, when CO_2 accumulates in the body (primary event), kidneys retain HCO_3 (compensatory) and along with buffers normalize the pH in 3-5 days.

So, the clinical picture of acid-base disturbances may show either one of the three stages.

- Acute stage (where either HCO_3 or $PaCO_2$ is altered with altered pH).
- Partially compensated stage (where both HCO_3 and $PaCO_2$ are altered with altered pH).
- Fully compensated (where both HCO_3 and $PaCO_2$ are altered with near normal pH).

METABOLIC ACIDOSIS

This is the commonest acid-base disorder. Effective management of metabolic acidosis needs anion gap calculation. Anion gap helps to categorize metabolic acidosis into two broad groups. Metabolic acidosis with increased anion gap (normochloremic acidosis) and metabolic acidosis with normal anion gap (hyperchloremic acidosis).

Anion Gap

A small amount of anion that cannot be measured by biochemical investigations is named as anion gap.

$(Na^+ + K^+) = (Cl + HCO_3) + (\text{unmeasured anions})$

(Anion gap)

$(135 + 04) = (100 + 24) + 8 \text{ to } 16$

If increased anion gap acidosis is evident the etiology should be identified and corrected where administration of HCO_3 may be hazardous. In children with normal anion gap acidosis (hyperchloremic acidosis) bicarbonate correction should be done judiciously.

Since acidosis is beneficial to the body homeostasis, correction should be attempted only when HCO_3 goes below 15 mEq/L (pH 7.2 or base deficit reaches 10 mmol/L). Overzealous correction of acidosis with HCO_3 leads to adverse effects like shifting of oxygen hemoglobin dissociation curve to the left resulting in poor release of oxygen at tissue level, precipitation of hypokalemia, intraventricular hemorrhage, hypernatremia and hypocalcemic tetany. So, the correction of acidosis is advised only when HCO_3 falls below 15 mEq/L.

(15-measured HCO_3) × 0.3 × body weight (in kg). Half of the HCO_3 correction can be done immediately by slow intravenous administration after diluting with 5% dextrose, the rest can be added in the maintenance fluid over 24 hours.

METABOLIC ALKALOSIS

Metabolic alkalosis results due to loss of acids (H^+ ions) from the gastrointestinal tract, through renal mechanisms, due to alkali gain or due to disproportionate loss of extracellular fluid.

Estimation of urinary chloride may help to differentiate saline responsive (urine chloride level < 10 mEq/L) from saline resistant (urine chloride >10 mEq/L) type of metabolic alkalosis.

Saline responsive metabolic alkalosis is managed by maintaining adequate ECF volume and serum potassium.

Metabolic alkalosis resulting from increased aldosterone activity (saline resistant) will respond to aldosterone antagonists (spiranolactone), ACE inhibitors or amiloride.

ABG Symbols and Values

Tem	*Symbol*	*Normal value*	*Range*	*Unit*
H^+	H^+	40	36-44	Nmol/L
pH	pH	7.4	7.36-7.44	–
CO_2 tension	$PaCO_2$	40	36-44	mm Hg
Base excess	BE	0	– 2 to +2	mmol/L
Total CO_2	TCO_2	25	23-27	mmol/L
Actual HCO_3	HCO_3	24	22-26	mmol/L
Standard HCO_3	SBC	24	22-26	mmol/L
O_2 saturation	SaO_2	98	95-100	%
O_2 tension	PaO_2	95	80-100	mm Hg

RESPIRATORY ALKALOSIS

Mild respiratory disorders causes hypoxemia (oxygenation failure or type I respiratory failure) resulting in respiratory alkalosis. The hypoxic drive causes hyperventilation and wasting out of CO_2. Other than lung diseases, heart disease, sepsis, CNS infection and hysterical over breathing may result in respiratory alkalosis. Children with respiratory alkalosis need prompt oxygen supplementation (6-8 lit/min) apart from correcting the basic pathological condition. Respiratory alkalosis induced by hysterical breathing is managed by rebreathing in paperbag.

RESPIRATORY ACIDOSIS

Advanced respiratory disease, thoracic cage and neuromuscular dysfunction leads to CO_2 retention ($PaCO_2$ > 45 mm of Hg) resulting in respiratory acidosis also known as ventilatory (type II) failure. In ventilatory failure CO_2 should be eliminated from the body by mechanical ventilatory support.

Arterial Blood Gas (ABG) Specimen Collection

The radial artery at the wrist is the most preferred site of ABG specimen collection. The other sites used are poplitial, brachial or femoral.

The injection site is cleaned with iodine or alcohol. Heparinized syringe with 22 gauge needle should be held like a pen with 45° angle and the artery should be punctured just 2 cm above the wrist crease.

- Ensure an adequate sample; avoid bubbles-dead space in the syringe will allow CO_2 and O_2 to diffuse in or out of the sample. Seal the syringe with a plastic cap for the same reasons.
- Avoid excess heparin. Fill the dead space of a ml syringe and attached needle with 1/1000 heaprin. A pre-heparinized syringe is preferable. 0.05 ml of heparin is enough for 1 ml of blood, upto 0.1 ml of heparin may interfere with blood gas values.
- Minimize metabolism in the sample. Delay in analysis allows O_2 consumption and CO_2 generation. If delay of more than a few minutes is anticipated store the sample on ice.

ASTERIAL BLOOD GAS INTERPRETATION

Step 1: Assess the pH. If it is raised > 7.44 suggests alkalosis or lowered < 7.36 suggests acidosis. This is the overall status of the patient.

Step 2:

	Acidosis	*Alkalosis*
Respiratory	CO_2 ↑	CO_2 ↓
Metabolic	Base excess ↓ or Bicarbonate ↓	Base excess ↑ or Bicarbonate ↑

Look at the CO_2 on the chart above.

- If the CO_2 agrees with the pH, i.e. low pH agrees with high CO_2 (acidosis) and high pH agrees with low CO_2 (alkalosis), then the overall picture is a respiratory acidosis or alkalosis.
- If the CO_2 disagrees with the pH, it is compensating for a metabolic abnormality.

Step 3: Confirm your findings by looking at the base excess and bicarbonate.

- If the base excess agrees with the pH, i.e. low pH with negative base excess (acidosis), the overall picture is a metabolic acidosis or alkalosis.
- If the base excess disagrees with the pH, it is compensating for a respiratory abnormality.

Example

In a patient with shock, showing sighing respiration

pH	7.24
PCO_2	31
HCO_3	14
BE	–18

- The pH is low, showing acidosis
- The pCO_2 disagrees with the pH (a low CO_2 indicates respiratory alkalosis, not an acidosis). Therefore it is compensating for metabolic acidosis.
- The base excess agrees with the pH (A negative base excess indicates a metabolic acidosis).

- Therefore, the patient is acidotic. Patient has a metabolic acidosis, which is being partially compensated by a respiratory alkalosis.

Step 4:

Oxygen Status

While accessing the oxygenation status, knowledge regarding age of the child and the inspired, oxygen concentration (FiO_2) are very important. The normal value of PaO_2 is 80-100 mm of Hg, in children and adults. $PaO_2 = FiO_2 \times 5$.

Step 5:

Simple or Mixed Disorder

In simple acid base disorder, both $PaCO_2$ and HCO_3 change in the same direction. If they do not follow this trend, the possibility of mixed disorder is likely. If the difference between total CO_2 (TCO_2) and HCO_3 is more than 1.2 in addition to metabolic problems, the underlying respiratory disturbance should be thought off. When both actual bicarbonate and standard bicarbonate are not the same, in addition to respiratory added metabolic component should be thought off. Common problems leading on to mixed disturbance are acute severe asthma, shock, cardiopulmonary arrest, respiratory distress syndrome in newborn, salicylate poisoning and diuretic therapy.

Step 6:

Acute or Chronic Problem

By knowing the duration of illness, we can tell whether it is an acute or a chronic problem. This knowledge is important because the compensation that occurs during acute and chronic stage especially in respiratory disorders grossly differs due to delayed renal compensation that occurs in addition to buffer base adjustment.

Step 7:

Laboratory Error

According to the Henderson-Hasselbach equation, out of the three measured values. (pH, $PaCO_2$, HCO_3) if two are known, the third can be calculated. It is also used to verify whether the three given values are mutually compatible.

Sometimes the bicarbonate values reported with the electrolytes will not tally with the ABG bicarbonate. Doubt arises about which value is correct. In such cases check the blood pH by using the formula

$$H = \frac{24 \times PCO_3}{HCO_3}$$

(pH is presented as H^+ ion concentration)

For example, If S bicarbonate level = 15 mEq/L and blood gas bicarbonate is 20 mEq/L pH 7, 40, PCO_2 is 33. Calculate the value closer to pH using the above formula.

$$H = \frac{24 \times 33}{15} = 52$$

$$H = \frac{24 \times 33}{20} = 40$$

Hence, the latter is nearer to the pH.

pH : Estimated (H^+)

Estimation of H^+ from pH:

pH	Estimated (H^+)
7.0	98
7.10	78
7.20	63
7.30	50
7.40	40
7.50	32
7.60	26
7.70	20

CAUSES OF METABOLIC ACIDOSIS

Increased anion gap (Normochloremic acidosis)	*Normal anion gap (Hyperchloremic acidosis)*
Lactic acidosis	Diarrhea
Shock	Renal tubular acidosis
Asphyxia	Uretro sigmoidostomy
Cyanide poisoning	Parenteral alimentation
Salicylate poisoning	Rapid ECF expansion
Paraldehyde poisoning	Exogenous chlorides
Biguanides poisoning	$CaCl_2$, $MgCl_2$, NH_4Cl
Organic acidemias	Cholestyramine
Inborn errors of carbohydrate and pyruvate metabolism	Carbolic anhydrase inhibitors
	Small bowel/biliary fistula

Ketoacids
  Diabetes mellitus
  Starvation
Sulphuric/phosphoric acid
  Renal failure

ABG DISORDER-EXPECTED COMPENSATION

Disorder	*Compensation*
Metabolic acidosis (HCO_3)	For every 1 mEq/L fall in HCO_3 $PaCO_2$ should Fall by 1 mm of Hg (1-1.5)
Metabolic alkalosis (HCO_3)	For every 1 mEq/L increase HCO_3 $PaCO_2$ should increase by 1 mm of Hg (0.5-1)
Respiratory acidosis ($PaCO_2$)	
Acute	For every 1 mm ↑ $PaCO_2$, HCO_3 ↑ by 0.2 mEq
Chronic	For every 1mm ↑ $PaCO_2$, HCO_3↑ by 0.4 mEq.
Respiratory alkalosis ($PaCO_2$)	
Acute	For every 1mm ↓ $PaCO_2$, HCO_3 ↓ by 0.2 mEq
Chronic	For every 1mm ↓ $PaCO_2$, HCO_3 ↓ by 0.5 mEq

37

Respiratory Failure

History should consider following points. Does the patient have factors that increase the risk for respiratory failure? Factors may include young age; history of prematurity; immunodeficiency; and chronic pulmonary, cardiac, or neuromuscular disease. History suggestive of an etiology like upper respiratory symptoms, fever, sedative exposure or neuromuscular weakness.

Physical

During physical examination, clinicians should avoid interfering with the patient's mechanisms for compensation. Children often find the most advantageous position for breathing. Children with respiratory distress commonly sit up and lean forward to improve leverage for the accessory muscles and to allow for easy diaphragmatic movement. Children with epiglottitis sit upright with their necks extended and heads forward while drooling and breathing through their mouths. Making a child lie down or making him or her cry during an otoscopic examination can precipitate acute respiratory failure.

General Appearance

Does the patient appear well or sick? Is the patient cyanotic?

- Respiratory rate, quality, and effort
  - Bradypnea is most often observed in central control abnormalities.

- The fast and shallow breathing of tachypnea is most efficient in intrathoracic airway obstruction.
- Auscultation provides information about the symmetry and quality of air movement. Evaluate the patient for stridor, wheezing, crackles, and decreased breath sounds and grunting.

- Assess for accessory muscle use and nasal flaring. Evaluate for paradoxical movement of the chest wall.
  - Tachycardia and hypertension may occur.
  - Patients may be lethargic, irritable, anxious, or unable to concentrate.

Causes

The most common reasons for respiratory failure in the pediatric population are divided into anatomic compartments, as follows:

- *Extrathoracic airway*:
  - Acquired lesions like retropharyngeal abscess, traumatic causes congenital lesions like subglottic stenosis, subglottic web or cyst
- *Intrathoracic airway and lung*:
  - Acute respiratory distress syndrome (ARDS), asthma
  - *Respiratory pump*: Chest wall abnormality or respiratory muscle failure.
- Central causes like CNS infection

Lab Studies

- An arterial blood gas can be used to define acute respiratory failure. Arbitrary definitions include a $PaCO_2$ greater than 50 mm Hg, a PaO_2 less than 60 mm Hg, or arterial oxygen saturation less than 90%.
- An elevated serum bicarbonate level suggests metabolic compensation for chronic hypercapnia.
- A complete blood cell count may be helpful; polycythemia suggests chronic hypoxemia.
- Electrolyte abnormalities can contribute to weakness; hypokalemia, hypocalcemia, and hypophosphatemia can impair muscle contraction.
  - Calculate the alveolar-arterial oxygen difference ($[A\text{-}a]DO_2$), which is the difference between the alveolar partial pressure

of oxygen (PAO < SUB < 2) and PaO_2. This value is an index of the efficiency of gas exchange by the lungs.

Medical Care

Management of acute respiratory failure begins with a determination of the underlying etiology. While supporting the respiratory system and ensuring adequate oxygen delivery to the tissues, initiate an intervention specifically defined to correct the underlying condition. For example, a patient with status asthmaticus is given supplemental oxygen to treat hypoxemia, but corticosteroids and beta-agonist drugs are also given to treat the underlying pathology.

Extrathoracic Airway Support

- For partial upper-airway obstruction, place a nasopharyngeal airway to provide a passageway for air; for example, obstruction caused by anesthesia or acute tonsillitis.
- An oropharyngeal airway can be used temporarily in the unconscious patient.
- For extrathoracic airway obstruction, such as croup, the following measures may be helpful:
  - Inspired humidity to liquefy secretions
  - Heliox (helium and oxygen gas mixture) to decrease work of breathing: A helium concentration of 60-80% has a density lower than that of air and improves breathing by reducing turbulent airflow through a narrowed area. A requirement for inspired oxygen (> 0.4) is a limiting factor in the use of Heliox.
  - Racemic epinephrine 2.25%, an aerosolized vasoconstrictor.
  - Systemic corticosteroids to decrease airway edema.
- Instrumentation with an endotracheal tube is occasionally needed to maintain its patency in certain cases (e.g. epiglottitis, thermal burns to the airway, severe croup).

Tracheal Intubation

- In general, uncuffed tubes are used in children younger than 8 years because the subglottic trachea surrounded by the cricoid cartilage is the narrowest part of the pediatric airway.

- In neonates and infants younger than 6 months, an endotracheal tube with an inner diameter (ID) of 3 or 3.5 mm is appropriate.
- In infants aged 6-12 months, a tube with a 3.5 or 4 mm ID is appropriate.
- In children older than 1 year, the following formula can be used: Tube size (ID in millimeters) = (age in years + 16)/4

Lung and Respiratory Pump Support

- *Oxygen therapy*
  - The initial treatment for hypoxemia is to provide supplemental oxygen.
  - High-flow (> 5-6 L/min) oxygen delivery systems include a Venturi-type device that places an adjustable aperture lateral to the stream of oxygen. Oxygen is mixed with entrained room air, and the amount of air is adjusted by varying the aperture size. The oxygen hoods and tents also supply high gas flows.
  - Low-flow (< 6 L/min) oxygen delivery systems include the nasal cannula and simple facemask.

Continuous Positive Airway Pressure (CPAP)

- CPAP may be indicated if lung disease results in severe oxygenation abnormalities such that an FiO_2 greater than 0.6 is needed to maintain a PaO_2 greater than 60 mm Hg.
- CPAP in pressures from 3-10 cm H_2O is applied to increase lung volume and may redistribute pulmonary edema fluid from the alveoli to the interstitium.
- CPAP enhances ventilation to areas with low V/Q ratios and improves respiratory mechanics.
- If a high concentration of FiO_2 is needed and if the patient does not tolerate even short periods of discontinued airway pressure, positive-pressure ventilation should be administered.

Noninvasive Positive Pressure Ventilation (NPPV)

- Noninvasive mechanical ventilation refers to assisted ventilation provided with nasal prongs or a facemask instead of an endotracheal or tracheostomy tube.

- This therapy can be administered to decrease the work of breathing and to provide adequate gas exchange.
- NPPV can be given by using a volume ventilator, a pressure-controlled ventilator, or a device for bilevel positive airway pressure (BIPAP or bilevel ventilator).
- The severity of the patient's disease limits the use of this technique if periodic relief from the facemask or nasal prongs is unavailable for days. A tracheal tube is necessary and safer under these circumstances.

Conventional Mechanical Ventilation

- Mechanical ventilation increases minute ventilation and decreases deadspace. This approach is the mainstay of treatment for acute hypercapnia and severe hypoxemia.
- A primary strategy for mechanical ventilation should be the avoidance of high-peak inspiratory pressures and the optimization of lung recruitment.
- Conventional mechanical ventilation optimizes lung recruitment, increases mean airway pressure and functional residual capacity, and reduces atelectasis between breaths.

Nonconventional Modes of Ventilation

- *Inverse ratio ventilation*
  - During positive pressure ventilation, the inspiratory phase is prolonged in excess of the expiratory phase.
  - It increases mean airway pressure and improves oxygenation during severe acute lung disease.
  - It is a nonphysiologic pattern for breathing; therefore, these patients are administered heavy sedation and paralysis.

Airway Pressure Release Ventilation (APRV)

APRV is a relatively new form of inverse-ratio ventilation in which a continuous gas flow circuit is used. This method allows the patient to breathe spontaneously throughout the ventilatory cycle.

High Frequency Oscillatory Ventilation (HFOV)

- HFOV combines small tidal volumes (smaller than the calculated airway dead space) with frequencies of >1 Hz to minimize the effects of elevated peak and mean airway pressures.

- HFOV has proven benefit in improving the occurrence and treatment of air-leak syndromes associated with neonatal and pediatric acute lung injury.

Adjunctive Therapies for Severe Hypoxemia

Inhaled nitric oxide (NO)

- NO is an endogenous free radical that mediates smooth muscle relaxation throughout the body. When delivered by means of inhalation, the potential benefit of NO is to improve ventilation

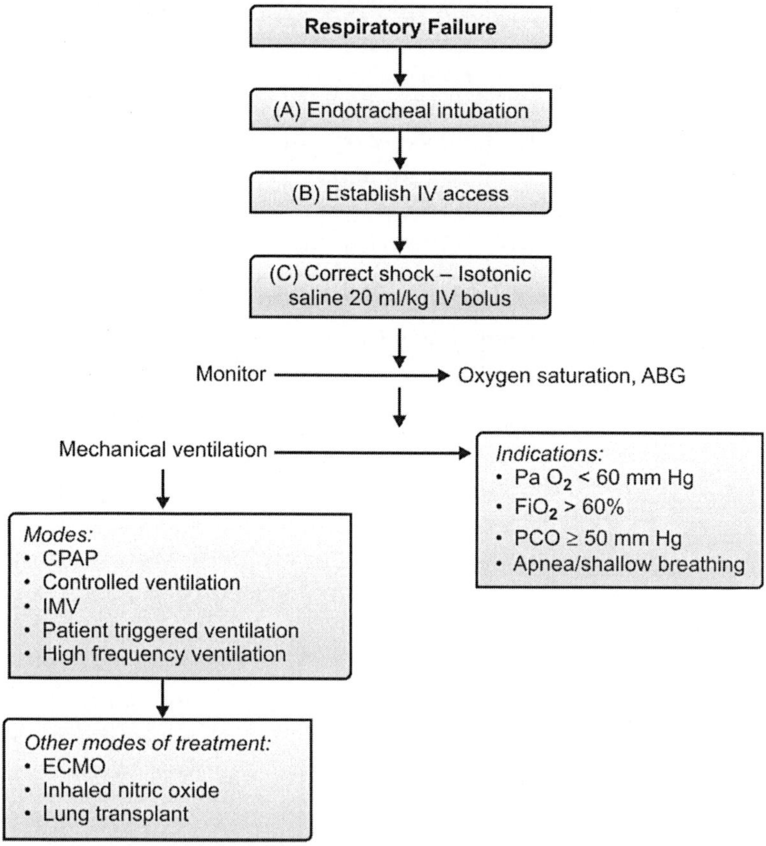

Note: If upper airway obstruction – Tracheostomy
If foreign body is present – Bronchoscopy

to perfusion matching by enhancing pulmonary blood flow to well-ventilated parts of the lung.
- This therapy is relatively safe because hemoglobin inactivates it quickly and does not cause systemic vasodilation leading to hypotension.

Administration of Exogenous Surfactant

- Relative surfactant deficiency is variably present as a consequence of many lung diseases.
- Exogenous surfactant replacement is of clear benefit to improve respiratory mechanics and oxygenation in the neonatal respiratory distress syndrome (RDS). Its role in severe lung injury in other pediatric populations is still investigated.

Rescue Therapy with Extracorporeal Life Support (ECLS)

- ECLS: blood is removed from the patient, passed through an artificial membrane where gas exchange occurs, and is returned to the body by either the arterial (venoarterial [VA]) or venous (venovenous [VV]) system.
- VV ECLS has become the preferred method for patients of all age groups who do not require cardiac support.

DIAGNOSTIC CRITERIA

Clinical

- Marked wheezing
- Progressive dyspnea
- Reduced breath sounds
- Cyanosis inspite of oxygen inhalation
- Pulsus paradoxus >15 mm of Hg.
- Marked restlessness
- Tachypnea/Bradypnea/Apnea/Grunting
- Weak or absent
  - cough reflex
  - Gag reflex
  - Pooled oropharyngeal secretion

Laboratory

- $PaO_2 < 60$ mm Hg (Breathing room air)
  $PaO_2 < 100$ mm Hg (Breathing 100% O_2)
- $PaCO_2 > 50$ mm Hg
- $pH < 7.3$

Appendix

DRUGS IN RESUSCITATION

Drug	*Indication*	*Dose*	*Route*	*Response*	*Complication*
Sodium (4.2%) 0.5 mEq/ml	Metabolic acidosis	2-3 mEq/ kg/ dose	IV over 2-5 min	Increased pH if adequately ventilated	Hypernatremia, Hyperosmolar solution, risk for IVH
Epinephrine (1:10,000)	Asystole or severe bradycardia	0.1-0.2 ml/kg	IV,ETT	Increased heart rate, BP and cardiac output	Hypertension, ventricular fibrillation
Glucose (10%)	Hypoglycemia	0.5 g/kg (5 ml/kg) followed by infusion 5 ml/kg/hr (Approx 8 mg/kg/min)	IV	Increases blood glucose	
Glucose (25%)	Hypoglycemia	0.5 g/kg (2 ml/kg)	IV	Increased blood glucose	Rebound hypoglycemia, hyperosmolar solution
Calcium Gluconate (10%)	Low cardiac output	1-2 ml/kg dose	IV over 2-5 minutes	Improved cardiac output	Bradycardia, dysarrhythmias
Dopamine	Low cardiac output, shock	5-20 mg/kg/ min to maintain BP	IV	Increased cardiac output,	Dysarrhythmias Decrease renal perfusion at rate >12-15 mg/ kg/min
Volume expanders: Albumin 5% Fresh frozen plasma (1 g/20 ml)	Hypovolemic shock	10-20 ml/kg (0.5-1g/kg)	IV over 2-4 hrs	Increased perfusion	Circulatory overload in cardiogenic shock. Contains 0.13-0.16 mEq Na/ml
Naloxone (Narcan 0.4 mg/ml)	Narcotic depression (rare)	0.2 mg/kg/dose (0.5 ml/kg) 0.01 mg/kg/ dose for reversal of opiate analgesia	IV, ET IM, SC	Improved respiratory effort when given rapidly repeat prn	Respiratory depression at birth, when mother was given narcotics prior to delivery.
Atropine	Bradycardia even after epinephrine	0.01 mg/kg/dose (0.025 ml/kg/ dose)	IV	Normal HR	Hyperthermia, tachycardia urinary retention.

INTUBATION SEDATION GUIDELINES

Drug Name	*Standard Dosage per Weight*	*Route*	*Special Considerations*
Atropine	0.02 mg/kg	IV	Do not use if < 2 kg Infuse over 1 min. Minimum dose 0.1 mg/dose
Midazolam	0.05-0.1 mg/kg 0.2–0.3 mg/kg	IV Intranasally	Do not use if < 35 weeks gestational age Do not use if < 35 weeks gestational age.
Fentanyl	1-4 mcg/kg	IV	Infuse slow IV push Have Pancuronium 0.1 mg/kg IV 1 at bedside
Muscle Relaxants – Only use if able to provide adequate Facial/Mask PPV			
Succinylcholine	1-2 mg/kg	IV	Use 2 mg/kg/dose if <1 year always administer atropine first. Do not repeat dose
Rocuronium	0.6-1.2 mg/kg	IV	
Vecuronium (Norcuron)	0.1 mg/kg	IV	Dilute dry powder 10 mg vial with 10 ml of NS or sterile water for injection. Preferred paralytic for neonates if necessary
Pancuronium (Pavulon)	0.1 mg/kg		

INOTROPIC AND VASOACTIVE AGENTS COMMONLY USED IN SHOCK

Drug	*Dose (μg/kg/min)*	*Hemodynamic Effect*	*Comment*
Dopamine	1-5	Splanchnic, renal and cerebral vasodilatation	Stimulates beta receptors by direct and indirect mechanisms; may cause tachydysrhythmias; doses >20 μg/kg/min occasionally required for normotension, but may result in severe tissue ischemia.
	5-15	Increased contractility and heart rate	
	15-20	Peripheral and renal vasoconstriction	
Dobutamine	1-20	Increased contractility	Minimal effect on heart rate; no selective renal effect
Isoproterenol	0.05-0.5	Increased contractility and heart rate; peripheral vasodilatation	May cause tachydysrhythmias; increases myocardial oxygen consumption
Epinephrine	0.05-1.0	Increased contractility and heart rate; marked peripheral, renal and mesenteric vasoconstriction	May cause tachydysrhythmias; increases myocardial oxygen consumption; increases glucose levels; increased risk of severe tissue ischemia.
Norepinephrine	0.05-1.0	Marked peripheral vasoconstriction	May cause severe tissue and organ ischemia; use in combination with vasodilator
Nitroprusside	0.05-8.0	Peripheral arterial and venous vasodilatation	Risk of cyanide toxicity
Hydralazine	0.1-0.5 mg/kg q3-6 h	Peripheral arterial vasodilatation	May produce reflex tachycardia

STANDARD IV INFUSION

1. *Adenosine*
   Injection – 6 mg/2 ml
   Diluent – NS
   1 ml of Adenosine (3 mg) + 5 ml NS
   6 ml = 3000 mcg pH 6.3-7.3
   1 ml = 500 mcg
   0.1 ml = 50 mcg
   Infuse as 0.1 ml (50 mgm)/kg/dose over 2 seconds

2. *Adrenaline*
   Injection – 1 mg/ml (1:1000)
   Diluent – NS, G5%, G10%
   To prepare standard infusion of 50 mcg/ml
   Adrenaline 1 ml = 1mg
   Add 1 ml adrenaline + 19 ml NS, G5%, G10%
   1 mg in 20 ml
   1000 micro gm in 20 ml
   100 mcg in 2 ml, 50 mcg/ml
   Compatible – Heparin, Dobutamine, Doxapram
   Incompatible – Aminophyllin, Lignocaine, Sod. Bicarbonate
   pH– 2.5-3.6
   Protect infusion from sunlight

3. *Aminophylline*
   Injection 250 mg/10 ml
   Diluent NS, G5%, G10%
   250 mg in 10 ml
   1 ml Aminophylline (25 mg) + 4ml of NS, G5%, G10%
   5 ml = 25 mg
   1 ml = 5 mg
   Compatible – Heparin, Dopamine
   Incompatible – Adrenalin, Amiodarone, Cefotaxime, Dobutamine, Doxapram, Insulin, Morphine
   pH 8.5 – 10.0

4. *Alprostadil (Prostaglandin E1)*
   Injection 500 mcg/ml or 0.5 mg/ml
   Diluent – NS, G5%

To prepare a standard infusion of 5 mcg/ml
(i.e. 5000 nano grams in 1 ml)
Babies under 1 kg
Draw 0.5 ml Alprostadil (500 mcg/ml) and add to
49.5 ml of NS or G 5%
50 ml = 250 micrograms
1 ml = 5 micrograms = 5000 nanograms
To prepare a standard infusion of 10 microgram/ml
(i.e. 10,000 nanograms in 1 ml)
Babies over 1 kg weight.
Draw 1 ml Alprostadil (500 microgram) and add to 49 ml NS or G5% and mix well.
50 ml = 500 micrograms
1 ml = 10 micrograms = 10000 nanograms

5. *Diazepam*
Injection 10 mg/2 ml
Diluent – G5% or G10%
To prepare standard solution of 0.1 mg/ml or
100 microgram/ml
Take 2 ml Diazepam (10 mg) + 98 ml G5% or G10%
100 ml = 10 mg
1 ml = 0.1 mg = 100 micrograms
Infuse as 50-100 µgm/kg/hour
Incompatible – Do not infuse with any other drug including NS
pH– 8.

6. *Doxapram*
Injection 100 mg/5 ml
Diluent – NS, G5%, G10%
To prepare standard infusion of 1000 microgram in 1 ml
Take 2.5 ml Doxapram injection (50 mg)
+ 47.5 ml of NS, G5% or G10%
50 ml = 50 mg
1 ml = 1 mg = 1000 micrograms
Compatible – Adrenaline, Dopamine, KCl, Salbutamol
Incompatible – Alkaline solutions, i.e. Aminophyllin, digoxin
Furosemide, thiopentone.

7. *Digoxin*
   Elixir 50 microgram = 0.05 mg/ml
   Injection 100 microgm = 0.1 mg in 1 ml
   Diluent – NS or G5%
   Take 1 ml of digoxin injection (100 micrograms)
   + 4 ml of NS or G5%
   5 ml = 100 microgram
   1 ml = 20 microgram
   Compatible – Furosemide, Heparin, Lignocaine, Morphine, KCl, Verapamil.
   Incompatible – Dobutamine, Doxapram, Fluconazole.
   pH 6.8-7.2

8. *Dobutamine*
   Inj 250 mg/20 ml
   Diluent – NS, G5%, G10%
   To prepare a standard infusion of 1000 micrograms or 1 mg in 1 ml
   Dobutamine 250 mg/20 ml, i.e. 12.5 mg/ml
   Take Dobutamine 4 ml (250 mg in 20 ml) + 46 ml
   50 mg in 50 ml
   1 mg in 1ml
   1000 micrograms in 1 ml
   Compatible – Adrenaline, Amiodarone, Atropine, Dopamine, Isoprenaline, Hydralazine, Lignocaine, Morphine, Noradrenaline, Pethidine, Phentolamine, Propranolol, Streptokinase
   In compatible – Acyclovir, Alkalis, Aminophylline, digoxin, Furosemide, $MgSO_4$, Soda bicarb
   pH 2.5-5.5

9. *Dopamine*
   Injection 200 mg/5 ml
   Diluent – NS, G5%, g10%
   To prepare a standard infusion of 1,000 microgram in 1 ml
   Dopamine contains 200 mg in 5 ml, i.e. 40 mg in 1 ml
   Take 1 ml Dopamine + 39 ml NS, G5% or G10% and mix well
   40 mg in 40 ml
   1 mg = 1 ml
   1000 microgram in 1 ml

Compatible – Aminophylline, Amiodarone, Chloramphenicol Dobutamine, Doxapram, KCl, Streptokinase, Tolazoline
Incompatible – Acyclovir, Amphotericin, Benzyl penicillin Furosemide, Soda bicarb and other alkaline solutions.
pH 2.25 – 4.5

10. *Epoprostenol (Prostacycline)*
Injection = 500 microgram
Diluent – Diluent provided, NS
Reconstitute with diluent provided to make 500 micrograms in 50 ml.
10 microgram = 1 ml
10 microgram/ml – concentrated solution

A. *To prepare a standard infusion of 500 nanogram in 1 ml:*
For babies under 1 kg;
Take 2.5 ml of conc. solution (25 microgram) + 47.5 ml NS and mix well.
25 micrograms in 50 ml
500 nanograms in 1 ml

B. *To prepare a standard infusion of 1000 nanograms in 1 ml:*
For babies over 1 kg;
Take 5 ml of Conc. solution (50 micrograms) + 45 ml of NS mix well
50 ml = 50 micrograms
1 ml = 1 microgram
1 ml = 1000 nanograms
Incompatible – Do not infuse with any other drug including Glucose.
pH 10.5
50 ml = 100 microgram
1 ml = 2 microgram
0.1 ml = 0.2 microgram
Start with 0.2 mg/kg/min and increase to 2 mg/kg/min maximum
Compatible – Dobutamine, Heparin
pH 2.5-2.8

11. *Heparin*
Injection – 1000 units/ml
Diluent – NS, G5% or G10%

To prepare a standard infusion of 50 units in 1 ml
For small preterm babies
Take 2.5 ml of heparin (2500 units) + 47.5 ml of NS, G5% or G10% mix well.
2500 units in 50 ml
50 units in 1 ml.
To prepare a standard infusion of 100 units in 1 ml –
Larger babies and term babies
Take 5 ml of heparin (5000 units) + 45 ml NS, G5% or G10%, mix well.
5000 units in 50 ml
100 units in 1 ml
Compatible – Aminophylline, amphotericin, Ascorbic acid, Calcium gluconate, Digoxin, Isoprenaline, Noradrenaline, KCl, Streptokinase, Suxamethonium.
Incompatible – Most other drugs including antibiotics
Some antihistamines, narcotic analgesics, phenothiazines
pH 5-8.

12. *Insulin*
Insulin – 100 units/ml
Diluent – NS or water
To prepare a standard infusion of 0.1 unit in 1 ml
Take 1 ml of human neutral insulin (100 units)
+ 9 ml of NS or water mix well
100 units in 10 ml
10 unit in 1 ml
Take 0.5 ml of solution and add to 49.5 ml NS, G5% or 10% and mix
This gives 5 units in 50 ml
0.1 unit in 1 ml
Compatible – Heparin, Metoclopramide
Incompatible – Aminophylline, Phenytoin, Soda bicarb
Sulphonamides, Thiopentone
pH 7-7.8

DRUG FORMULATORY

Drug	*Route*	*Dosage*	*Comments*
Acetaminophen (crocin, calpol)	PO, PR	Newborn 25 mg/kg/d d/v 4-5 h Infant : 50-60 mg/kg/day d/v q4-6h	Contraindicated in infants with G-6PD deficiency. Overdose results in delayed hepatotoxicity. *Anti-dote*: N-acetyl cysteine. *Side effects*: hypokalemia, acidosis and GI disturbances
Alfacalcidol (1-a Vit D)	PO	0.05 µg/kg OD	
Albuterol	ET	0.05-0.15 mg/kg/dose q4-6h	Tachycardia, hypertension, arrhythmias, tremor, hypokalemia, irritability.
Atracurium (Tracrium)	IV	Loading: 0.5 mg/kg Maintenance: 5-10 mg/kg/day every 20-30 min (24 hrs after loading dose)	Indicated in infants requiring mechanical ventilation who continue to have inadequate oxygenation despite optimal supportive care. Has little effect on CVS.
Atropine (tropine) (600 µg/ml)	IV ET	0.01 mg/kg/dose, to be repeated q 10-15 minutes with the total maximum dose of 0.04 mg/kg	Indicated for bradycardia, presumed to be vagal in origin. *Side effects*: Dry mouth, blurred vision, hyperthermia, tachycardia, constipation, urinary retention, restlessness. *Contraindication*: Glaucoma, tachycardia. *Antidote*: Physostigmine
Budesonide 1 mg/2ml. MDI 200 µg puff	Nebulized	500 mg-1 mg/dose diluted to 4 ml with NS q12h. 200 mg-1 mg/ dose q12h	
Caffeine Citrate	PO	Loading : 20 mg/kg Maintenance: 5-10 mg/kg/day q 6h. Dose of caffeine base is ½ the above dose	Methylxanthine derivative, compared with aminophylline it is more potent CNS stimulator, has the same but milder side effects. Should monitor serum levels. Therapeutic level 8-25 µg/ml. Contraindication: Caffeine benzoate preparation has been associated with causation of kernicterus.
Calcium Gluconate (10%) Injection	IV	*Cardiac resuscitation*: 1-2 ml/kg/dose (over 10 minutes) Symptomatic hypocalcemia: 1-2 ml/kg by slow infusion over 30 minutes	Contains elemental Ca^{++} 100 mg/ml. Monitor closely for bradycardia, dysrhythmias and extravasation. (may cause tissue necrosis) Infusion rate not to exceed 20 mg Ca^{++}/kg/min. *Side effects*: Hypotension and bradycardia, associated with arrhythmias in digitalized patient, may precipitate when used with bicarbonate.

Cond...

Cond...

Drug	*Route*	*Dosage*	*Comments*
	PO	*Maintenance*:2-4 ml/kg/ day (200-400 mg/kg/day) mixed in compatible IV fluids Q6h 400-800 mg/ kg/ day (36-72 mg/ kg/ day elemental Ca^{++}) divided equally among feedings q6h. Start with 400 mg/ kg/ day (36 mg/ kg/day of elemental Ca^{++}) and increase gradually.	IV preparation can be given orally to supplement nutritional intake in preterm infants to a total intake of 150 mg/kg/day of elemental calcium, including content of feedings. Less irritating to GI tract than calcium chloride.
Calcium Polystyrene Sulfonate (Resonium calcium)	PR, PO	Acute hyperkalemia: 1 mg/kg/dose q6h as needed	1 g/kg decreases serum K^+ by 0.5-2.0 mmol/L. Preparation of 0.25 g/ml in 25% sorbitol should be used to prevent GI obstruction.
Chloralhydrate	PO PR	10-30 mg/kg/dose q6-8 hprn Recommended maximum dose 100 mg/kg/day	Can cause gastric irritation; laryngospasm if aspirated. Caution in preterm infants; Avoid large doses in severe cardiac disease. Contraindicated in severe hepatic/renal impairment.
Chloropromazine (emetil)	PO,IM	750 μg/kg/dose q6h Maximum dose is 1.5 mg/kg q6h	Used in treatment of opiate withdrawal to reduce threshold for seizures. Not for IV use
Clonazepam (lonazep, rivotril)	IV PO	100-200 μg/kg bolus over 30 min or 10-30 mg/kg/hr infusion. *Maintenance*: 25-50 mg/ day	Increased secretions
Chlorpheniramine (avil)	IV	250 μg/kg for anaphylaxis	
Chlorothiazide (ditide)	PO/IV Never IM	20-40 mg/kg/day d/v q12h	Dehydration and electrolyte (Na, Cl,K) imbalance. Use with caution in liver and severe renal disease.
Cimetidine (lock-2)	PO IV	*Preterm*: 4-8 mg/kg/day divided q12h Term neonates: 10 mg/kg/day divided q8h Infants: 10-20 mg/kg/day divided q6h	Use in neonates still experimental. Reduction of dosage required in renal dysfunction. Can cause CNS side effects, diarrhea, rash. Increases serum levels of some drugs.
Cisapride	PO	0.2-0.3 mg/kg/dose q6-8h 30 minutes before feed.	Stop 24h prior to pH study. Diarrhea.
Cromolyn	ET	20 mg/dose	Bronchospasm, cough, nasal pharyngeal congestion
Dexamethasone (dexona)	IM, IV, PO	Pre-extubation to decrease upper airway edema: 1.5 mg/kg/day d/v q8h. Cerebral edema: Initial dose	Side effects include hypertension, hyperglycemia, salt retention, adrenal suppression. May increase risk of infection. Consider steroid

Cond...

Cond...

Drug	*Route*	*Dosage*	*Comments*
		= 0.5-1.5 mg/kg; Maintenance 0.2-0.5 mg/kg/day Q6h. Anti inflammatory 0.025-0.05 mg/kg/dose q6-12h.	coverage for periods of stress after therapy and in intercurrent illness.
Diazepam (Valium)	IV	0.1-0.3 mg/kg/dose slow IV push over 2 minutes; repeat q5-10 min up to a total dose of 1.0 mg/kg *For status epilepticus*: Bolus 0.2 mg/kg IV, followed by 0.1-0.3 mg/kg/h as continuous infusion (dilute in D5W to 0.1mg/ml)	*Indication*: not used as a first line anticonvulsant. Short-term adjunctive therapy in status epilepticus. Risk of CNS and respiratory depression, hypotension and phlebitis. Contraindicated in hyperbilirubinemic neonates. Caution in glaucoma, shock and depression.
	PR	0.5 – 1.0 mg/kg; Parenteral preparation to be used with a syringe and catheter inserted into the rectum.	
Digoxin (digoxin, lanoxin)	IV, PO	Loading mg/kg/IV Maintenance Preterm 20 mg 1 μg/kg/day)IV Term 30 mg 4-6 μg d/v q12h >2 mo 40 mg 6-8 μg d/v q12h 10 μg d/v q12h *Note*: Above dosages are for CHF, producing levels of 0.5-2 mg/ml. Higher doses may be needed for treatment of arrhythmias.	• Loading dose is given in three divided doses (1/2, ¼) q8h. Start maintenance 24 hours after last digitalizing dose in preterm and 12 hours after in full-term neonates. • Maintenance dose is generally 25% of the total loading dose. • The PO dose is 25% more than the IV dose. Caution in renal failure; contradiction – ventricular dysrhythmias.
Dobutamine (dobutrex)	IV	2.5-15 μg/kg min (maximum 30 μg/kg/min) Calculation: same as dopamine. 6×wt(kg)=mg to be added to 100 ml D5W.yields 1 ml/hr=1mg/kg/min.	Acts directly on β_1 receptors to increase myocardiac contractility. No dopaminergic effect. Adverse effect: dysrhythmias, systemic hypertension. Preferred over dopamine in the neonate with shock, but without severe hypotension. Incompatible with alkaline solutions.
Domperidone (domstal)	PO	Gastroesophageal reflux in older infants: 0.3 μg/kg/dose 10-20 min before food.	Dopamine antagonist. Gastrointestinal prokinetic agent.In young infants extrapyramidal reactions may occur
Dopamine (dopaplus)	IV	*Constant IV infusion*: Initial 2-5 μg/kg/min increasing gradually	Dose-dependent pharmacological actions: Renal: 2-4 μg/kg/min IV.

Cond...

Cond...

Drug	*Route*	*Dosage*	*Comments*
		up to 30 μg/kg/min for Desired cardiac/ vascular effects Minimum dilution = 1.6 mg/ml In D5W or D10 W *Calculation*: mg/100 ml = wt(kg) x 6 x desired dose mg/kg/min) desired IV fluid rate (ml/hr)	Inotropic (b_1): 5-10 μg/kg/min IV. Vasoconstrictive (a): 10 μg/kg/min IV. Care must be exercised to prevent local infiltration since vaso-constrictive activity will lead to vasospasm and tissue necrosis. Inform physician.
Edrophonium hydrochloride (Tensilon)	IV	Test for myasthenia gravis: 0.1 mg single dose.	Keep resuscitation kit ready as it may precipitate cholinergic crisis, arrhythmia, bronchospasm. C/I in GI or GU obstruction or arrhythmias. *Antidote*: 0.01-0.04 mg/kg/dose of atropine.
Enalapril (vasotec)	PO IV	0.005-0.01 mg/kg/dose q8-24h; depending on BP 5-10 μg/kg/dose q8h-24h; administer over 5 min	Cardiopulmonary compromise, hyperkalemia, agranulocytosis. CI in renal artery stenosis. Decrease dose in renal failure.
Epinephrine (Racemic) for inhalation 2.25%	Via Nebulizer	0.25m/kg diluted to 3 ml with normal saline q 1-2h Max total dose 0.5 ml.	May be useful in neonatal apnea resistant to theophylline. Do not use if seizure disorder, increased blood pressure or in first 3 days of life.
Epinephrine (1:1, 000) (1mg/ml)	IV	0.1-0.5 μg/kg min (infusion) mix with D5W or D10W *Calculation*: Same as Dopamine 0.5-1 ml of 1:10000 as inotropic agent	To support in babies with true or relative hypotension. Produces an increase in heart rate and systolic blood pressure.
Ergocalciferol (calciferol)	PO	*Preterm*: 400-800 IU/day	Hypercalcemia, weakness, diarrhea,
Erythromycin	PO IV	3-5 mg/kg/dose q6h 3-5 mg/kg/dose q6h; infuse over 60 min.	 GI distress
Ethamsylate	IM, IV	12.5 mg/kg q6h (total of 16 doses)	To reduce risk of cerebral hemorrhage in preterm infant.
Exosurf	IT	5 ml/kg/dose q 12h for details see, specific protocol	Synthetic surfactant for the prophylaxis and treatment of hyaline membrane disease
Fentanyl citrate (Sublimaze)	IV, SC	*Pain/sedation*: Slow IV over 5 min: 1-2 μg/kg/dose. *Anesthesia*: Slow IV over 5 min: 20-75 μg/kg/dose Onset of action: 1-2 min *Peak action*: 10 min.	Adverse effects; respiratory depression and apnea, bradycardia, functional ileus. Tolerance develops rapidly to sedative and analgesic effects, necessitating increases in dosage.
Fludorocortisone (Floricot)	PO	Congenital adrenal *hyperplasia*: 0.05 to 0.2 mg once a day	Excessive therapy can cause hypertension C/I: CHF.

Cond...

Cond...

Drug	*Route*	*Dosage*	*Comments*
Folic acid (folvite)	PO	Hemolytic anemia: 0.25 mg/kg/day for 6 months. Dietary supplementation in preterm (<33 wks) 50 µg/day.	Normal serum level >4 ng/ml.
Folinic acid	PO	5 µg/dose twice a week in toxoplasmosis	Used along with pyrimethamine.
Furosemide (Lasix) (20 mg/2 ml)	PO IV, IM	Initial; 1 mg/kg/ dose q 24h in preterm, q12 h in full-term; Maximum single IV dose is 2 mg/kg (IV push over 2-3 min) Maximum rate of infusion: 0.5 mg/kg/min 1-4 mg/kg/ dose	Dehydration and electrolyte (Na, Cl, K) imbalances, ototoxicity, metabolic alkalosis, nephrocalcinosis, hyperuricemia and increased calcium excretion.
Gentian violet (1%)	Topical	Dilute to 0.5% solution 3-4 drops q8h-12h	Stains the part. Do not apply over face.
Glucagon (glucagons novo)	IM, IV	30 µg/kg 1M; may repeat prn to max. 1 mg 0.5-2 µg/day	Limited use in neonates. Helpful in hypoglycemia only if liver glycogen is available. Indicated in persistent hypoglycemia despite aggressive aggressive glucose infusion (>14 mg/kg min) or problem of fluid over load.
Heparin (hep)	IV	To keep indwelling lines open: 1 unit/ml in flushing and parenteral solutions. For heparinization : Initial dose; 50 units/kg/hr *Maintenance*: 20-25 units/kg hr as infusion.	During heparinization monitor baseline and subsequent coagulation studies; clotting time, PT, APTT. Dilute with D5W or 10 D10W. Bleeding, allergy, alopecia, thrombocytopenia. CT = 20-30 min, APTT=1.5-2.5 times control value before dose. *Antidote*: Protamine sulfate (1 mg per 100U heparine in previous 4 hours)
Hepatitis B Immune globulin (HBIG) (hepaglob)	IM	200 IU as soon after birth as possible (within 12 hours)	For prophylaxis in newborns whose mothers are hepatitis B antigen (HbsAg) positive
Hepatitis B (Recombinant vaccine)	IM	0.5 ml (10 mg administered within 7 days of birth and again at 1 and 6 months of age	Hepatitis B vaccine may be given at the same time as HBIG, but should be given at a separate site.
Hyaluronidase (hynidase)	SC	15 unit diluted in 1 ml of saline and infiltrate the affected area	Use to treat IV extravasation of certain drugs, but do not use for extravasation of alpha adrenergic blockers, e.g. Dopamine
Hydralazine (apresoline)	IV	Initial dose: 0.2 mg/kg q 4-6h prn as required for BP control. Dose may be	Causes direct relaxation of smooth muscle in peripheral vascular bed. May cause

Cond...

Cond...

Drug	*Route*	*Dosage*	*Comments*
		Gradually increased by 0.1 mg/kg/dose to max 2 mg/kg/dose. Given by slow IV push at rate not exceeding 0.2 mg/min.	tachycardia, SVT, diarrhea, emesis, Lupus like syndrome, agranulocytosis, decrease dosage in renal failure.
	PO	PO dose generally twice the effective IV dose	Oral bioavailability generally 50% that of IV route.
Hydrochloro thiazide (hydride)	PO	2-4 mg/kg/day d/v q 12h start with 1 mg/kg/ day and increase the dose by 1 mg kg/day every 2 days	Same as chlorothiazide
Hydrocortisone (efcorlin)	IV	For adrenal crisis: 25 mg IV bolus, followed by continuous infusion of 50-100 mg/m^2/24 hr until improvement occurs. Anti-inflammatory: 1-2.5 mg/kg/dose.	Wide variation in glucocorticoid requirements. Dose must be individualized. Can cause adrenal suppression, fluid and electrolyte disturbance, hypertension, hyperglycemia, increases susceptibility to infections.
	PO	Mantenance dose for congenital adrenal hyperplasia: 20-25 mg/ m^2/day divided tid	
	IV	For neonatal hypoglycemia: 1-2 mg/kg/dose q8h	Indicated in persistent hypoglycemia despite aggressive glucose infusion (>14 mg/kg min) or problem of fluid overload.
Immunoglobulins: Hepatitis Bi-immunoglobulin (HBIG0 (hepaglob) (200 IU/ml)	IM	Neonates born to HbsAg positive mothers: 100-200 IU soon after birth (atleast <5 days) *Booster dose*: 32-48IU/kg between 2 and 3 months after initial dose.	
Human normal immunoglobins (Bharglob) IM	IM	Immunotherapy: 10% 0.6 ml/kg; 16.5% 0.4 ml/kg. Prophylaxis of infections 10% 0.4 ml/kg: 16.5% 0.25 ml/kg	*Clinical Investigations*: Selective IgA deficiencies, hypersensitivity. SP for signs of anaphylactoid reactions.
Rabies immunoglobulin	IM	20 IU/kg. 1/2 the dose should be infiltrated in and around the wound & 1/2 administered IM	First dose of vaccination given at the same time but at a different site.
RSV immunoglobulin	IV	750 mg (15 ml) monthly during RSV season	
Tetanus immunoglobulin (TIG) (Tetglob)	IM, IT	Tetanus neonatorum: 500-10000 IU IM or 250 IU IT prophylaxis: 250-500 IU IM	Local pain, fever, flushing and chills may occur
Varicella – Zoster immunoglobulin (VZIG)	IM	250 mg	Indicated in any mother suffering from chickenpox upto 5 days earlier to 15 days after delivery.

Cond...

Cond...

Drug	*Route*	*Dosage*	*Comments*
Immuno-globulin (sandoglobulin)	IV	Replacement therapy for congenital or acquired antibody deficiency: 100-200 mg/kg q 2-4 weeks *Treatment*: 0.2 g/day over 3 hour for 4 days; *Term*: 0.4 g/day over 3 hours for 4 days	Can cause anaphylactoid and hypersensitivity reaction start infusion at very slow rate and increase slowly.
		For neonates with passive autoimmune thrombo-cytopenia : 0.5 g/kg/day for 5 days.	Reconstitute in 0.9% saline solution as a 5% solution and infuse over 12 hours on each of 2 consecutive days
Indomethacin (microcid)	IV	0-7 days: 0.2 mg/kg/dose at Hour 0 0.1mg/kg/dose at hour 12 0.1mg/kg/dose at hour 36	Adverse effects; renal dysfunction, platelet dysfunction, hypoglycemia. n. Close monitoring of serum concentrations of drugs and dosage adjustments may be required.
Insulin (Actrapid)	IV	Start with 0.05 unit/kg/hr as a continuous infusion. (Add 10 U/kg of insulin to 100 ml of 10% dextrose 1ml/kg/hr=0.1U/kg/hr). Titrate infusion to maintain blood glucose concentration.	1-Flush tubing with 50 ml of solution prior to infusion. 2-Connect with the shortest possible tubing 1 and 2 will reduce absorption loss and improve delivery.
Glucose/ insulin infusion		This combination produces 1 unit insulin/ 2 gm glucose. 0.1 unit/kg insulin with 4 ml/kg of 25% dextrose for hyper-kalemia.	
Ipratropium bromide (Ipravent)	Via nebulizer	*Inhalation solution*: 0.125 mg (0.5 ml) diluted to 2-3 ml with NS q6h. Can be mixed with salbutamol.	Not enough experience with neonates. Could be used as bronchodilator in infants with BPD.
Iron	PO	Treatment of Iron deficiency: 6 mg/kg/day elemental iron Prevention of iron deficiency: 3 mg/kg/ day elemental iron	Fer-in-sol delivers 2.5 mg elemental iron/0.1 ml • Wt (kg) x 4.5 x (desired Hb– patients Hb) = mg of Iron.
Isoprenaline	IV	0.1-0.5 μg/kg/min as infusion	For bradycardia and hypotension.
Isoproterenol	IV infusion	0.05-0.5 μg/kg/min	Dose dependent inotropic and vasodilator effect. Adjust rate of infusions to keep HR < 200/ min. SP in CHF .

Cond...

Cond...

Drug	*Route*	*Dosage*	*Comments*
Kayexalate	PO,PR	0.5-1.0 Gm/kg q2-6h PRN	Has delayed onset, electrolyte disturbances, alkalosis.
Labetalol	PO,IV	Bolus 0.25 mg/kg over 2min dose can be doubled and repeated every 10 min until desired clinical response or total dose of 4 mg/kg is reached. *Maintenance:* 0.25-1 mg/kg/dose q4h (IV) 1.5-2 mg/kg/dose q12h (PO) 0.25-1.5 mg/kg/h continuous infusion.	CI in CHF, heart block, sinus tachycardia. May cause bradycardia, edema and bronchospasm.
Lidocaine (Xylocaine)	IV	Ventricular arrhythmias: Initial dose: 0.5 mg/kg over 5 min. May repeat once after 5 min subsequent infusion: 10-50 μg/kg/min.	For short-term control of ventricular arrhythmias; may cause hypotension. Should be used in critical care areas only. Seizures, asystole, respiratory arrest is also known.
Lidocaine/ prilocaine cream (EMLA cream)	Topical	2-5 g/site for painful procedures.	To be applied 60 min prior to the procedure.
Lorazepam (calmese)	IV	Initial: 0.05 mg/kg/dose, repeat every 15 min PRN Maintenance; 0.05 mg/kg dose Q 6-8h PRN	May be useful in seizures refractory to phenobarbital and phenytoin. May cause respiratory depression. Injectable product may be given rectally.
Magnesium Sulfate 50% inj (4 mEq/ml) or (2 mmol/ml)	IV	For hypomagnesemia; 25- 50 mg $MgSO_4$/kg /dose : may repeat q6h for 3-4 doses *Maintenance*: 31.2 mg-62.5 mg $MgSO_4$/kg day	For IV use, the solution should be diluted to 1% add 1 ml 50% sulfate injection to 49 ml NS or sterile water) and the required dose infused over 1 hour. To be added to total IV fluid. Monitor for hypotension, respiratory depression. SP in renal insufficiency and neonates on digoxin. *Antidote*: Calcium gluconate.
Mannitol (20%)	IV	0.5-2.0 g/kg/dose over 20 mins.	For management of cerebral edema.
Midazolam	IV,IM	Loading dose 50 mg/kg when on ventilator Maintenance of 50-150 mg/ kg/hr	
$NaCl_2$ (3%)	IV	4 ml/kg for hyponatremic seizures	Hypernatremia
Naloxone (Narcan) 20 mg/ml	IM,IV,SC	10 mg/kg for narcotic overload. Once may be repeated PRN at 2-3 min interval.	
Nifedipine (Depin)	SL	1-2 mg/kg/day in four divided doses	Should be given SL not to be swallowed. severe

Cond...

Cond...

Drug	*Route*	*Dosage*	*Comments*
			hypotension, edema, flushing, tachycardia. SP in CHF
Nitroglycerine	IV	Start with 0.1 μg/kg/min. and titrate infusion rate to desired response. Max dose 5 μg/kg/min 1-2 μg/kg/min – decreases preload 3-5 μg/kg/min – decreases after load	The role of nitroglycerin therapy in the neonate is at present unclear. It may preferred over nitroprusside in the treatment of severe cardiac failure.
Nitroprusside (Prusside)	IV	Initial 0.25 μg/kg/min. Titrate infusion rate by doubling rate of infusion until desired or adverse effects are observed. Recommended maximum rate of infusion is 6 mg/kg min. For infusion dilute to a concentration of 100 μg/ml. Protect solution and line from light.	Indicated in refractory hypertension. Toxicity manifested by hypotension, reflex tachycardia, methemoglobinemia, cyanide toxicity. Acute withdrawal may precipitate hypertensive crisis. Monitor thiocyanate levels if used >48 hrs.
Norepinephrine (Levophed)	IV	0.01-2.0 μg/kg/min	Tachycardia, hypertension. Avoid arterial infusion.
Pancuronium (Pavulon)	IV	0-1 week: 0.03 mg/kg/dose 1-2 weeks: 0.06 mg/kg/dose 2-4 weeks: 0.09 mg/kg/dose Infuse slowly over 3.5 minutes: repeated as required q1-2h.	Indicated in infants requiring mechanical ventilation who continue to have inadequate oxygenation despite optimal supportive care. Can cause tachycardia. *Antidote*: Neostigmine with atropine/glycopyrrolate
Paraldehyde	IV	*Loading*: 3 ml/kg/hr (150 mg/kg/hr) of a 5% solution x 3 hours. *Maintenance*: 0.4 ml/kg/hr (20 mg/kg/hr) of 5% solution.	For IV administration, add 5 ml (5 g) to 100 ml NS or D5W to make a 5% solution. Administer via syringe pump with a glass syringe. IV tubing and syringe must be protected from light by wrapping. IV tubing (and syringe if plastic) should be replaced every 4 hours.
	PR	0.3 ml/kg/dose q 4-6 h prn dissolve dose in equal volume of olive oil prior to administration. Irregularly absorbed by rectal route.	*Adverse effects*: Pulmonary edema and hemorrhage, hypotension, local irritation. Routine use discourage except for treatment of status epilepticus resistant to initial therapy. C/I in pulmonary or hepatic disease.
Phenobarbitone (Gardenal)	IV IV, IM, PO	*Loading*: 20 mg/kg IV slowly (max rate of infusion 2 mg/kg/min) Maintenance: 3-5 mg/	Indication: Neonatal seizures. If seizures continue after the initial IV loading dose, additional doses of 10 mg/kg (spaced at

Cond...

Cond...

Drug	*Route*	*Dosage*	*Comments*
		kg/day (first dose given 24 hours after loading)	20-30 minute intervals) can be given, up to a total loading dose of 40 mg/kg (must ensure adequate respiratory control if using high-dose). Liver enzyme inducing dose: 2 mg/kg/day. Sedation, lethargy and hypert-sensitivity reactions. Drug levels increased with alkalosis. *Drug interactions*: Reduces serum levels of drugs.
Phenytoin (Dilantin)	IV	Neonatal seizures: Loading:20 mg/kg IV slowly (maximum rate of infusion 0.5 mg/kg/min)	Infusion in NS only. Rapid IV administration may cause hypotension and bradycardia. Indication; neonatal seizures refractory to Phenobarbitol *Adverse effects*: Drowsiness, behavioral changes hypersensitivity reactions.
Prednisolone (Wysolone)	PO	0.5 mg/kg q6h	
Quinidine (Natcardine)	PO	5-15 mg/kg day d/v q6h	For abolishing and preventing premature contractions of atrial, A-V junctional or ventricular origin. Useful adjunct to digoxin in atrial flutter and fibrillation C/I in complete A-V block.
Salbutamol (Ventorlin) (5 mg/ml solution)	via nebulizer	For weight <1kg = 1.00 mg/dose For weight >1kg = 2.00 mg/dose Diluted to 2-3 ml with normal saline q2-6h prn	Monitor cardiovascular status.
Succinylcholine (Scoline)	IV	1-2 mg/kg/dose	Premedicate the patient with atropine (0.03 mg/kg) it will increase the serum level of potassium.

Natural surfactant extracts (NSEs)

- Survanta

Dose: 100 mg of phospholipids, i.e. 4 ml/kg

- Surfactant –TA

Dose: 60-120 mg/kg (Higher dose of 120 mg/kg better results)

- Curosurf (Porcine lung extract)

Dose: 200 mg/kg initially, followed by 100 mg/kg at 12 and 24 hrs later

- CLSE (calf lung surfactant extracts)

Dose: 100 mg/kg initially and subsequently

- Beractant

Dose: 100 mg/kg initially and subsequently

- SF-RI

Dose: 50 mg/kg B wt initially and subsequently

- Human amniotic fluid extract (homologous)

Dose: 60 mg/kg initially and subsequently

Synthetic surfactants

- ALEC

(7:3 mixture of DPPC: PG dispersed in 1 ml saline)

Dose: 100 mg for premature 23-34 wks.

  – At birth first dose as pharyngeal insulin.
  – Next after 10 ml, 1 hr and 24 hrs.

- Exosurf neonatal

(108 mg phospholipids DPPC in 10 ml phials with 10 ml of solvent)

  – 5 ml /kg birth wt.
  – 2 doses of 5 ml/kg at 12 hrs interval are recommended for rescue therapy.
  – In reference to DPPC, the dose is 67.5 mg DPPC/kg birth weight.

Cond...

Cond...

Drug	*Route*	*Dosage*	*Comments*
Terbutaline	PO SC	100 μg/kg/day 0.005-0.01 mg/kg/dose	For bronchospasm in BPD monitor heart rate.
Valproic acid	PO	Preterm: 15 μg/kg/day once daily full term: 40 mg/kg/day once daily. Can be increased upto 30 mg/kg/dose q 12hr	Dosage recommendations in neonates based on preliminary data. Its use should be restricted to infants with seizures refractory to more traditional therapy. *Adverse effects*: hepatoxicity (monitor serum transaminases), hyperammonemia. GI disturbances, sedation, altered coagulation, pancreatitis, Therapeutic serum levels; 350-700 μmol/L.
Vasopressin (aqueous)	IM, SC	2.5-10 U total dose q12h-q16h	Broncho constriction, diarrhea and electrolyte imbalance.
Multivitamin preparation in NICU	PO	1.6 ml per day	Contains (in 1.6 ml): Vitamin solution 1.0 ml Aquasol E (25. I.U) 0.5 ml Folic acid (0.05 mg 0.1ml Solution very hyperosmolar and should be diluted in at least four times the volume of formula for administration.

Index